ADVANCES IN SURGERY®
VOLUME 18

ADVANCES IN SURGERY®

VOLUME 15

VOLUME 16

VOLUME 17

ADVANCES *in* SURGERY®

VOLUME 18 • 1984

YEAR BOOK MEDICAL PUBLISHERS • INC.

CHICAGO

Library of Congress Catalog Card Number: 65-29931

International Standard Serial Number: 0065-3411

International Standard Book Number: 0-8151-7665-1

Contributors

JUAN BASS, M.D.
Division of General Surgery, University of Ottawa General Hospital, Ottawa, Ontario, Canada.

OLIVER H. BEAHRS, M.D.
The Section of Colon & Rectal Surgery, Mayo Clinic, Rochester, Minnesota.

HENRY BUCHWALD, M.D., PH.D.
Department of Surgery, University of Minnesota, Minneapolis, Minnesota.

P. T. CAHILL, M.D.
The New York Hospital-Cornell Medical Center, New York, New York.

E. STANLEY CRAWFORD, M.D.
Department of Surgery, Baylor College of Medicine and the Surgical Service of the Methodist Hospital, Houston, Texas.

JOHN M. DALY, M.D., F.A.C.S.
Associate Attending Surgeon, Department of Surgery, Memorial Sloan-Kettering Cancer Center; and Associate Professor of Surgery, Department of Surgery, Cornell University Medical College, New York, New York

JEROME J. DECOSSE, M.D., F.A.C.S.
Chairman, Department of Surgery, Memorial Sloan-Kettering Cancer Center; and Chairman, Department of Surgery, Cornell University Medical College, New York, New York.

JOEL B. FREEMAN, M.D., F.R.C.S.(c), F.A.C.S.
Division of General Surgery, University of Ottawa, Ottawa General Hospital, Ottawa, Ontario, Canada.

CLEON GOODWIN, M.D.
Department of Surgery, Cornell University Medical Center, New York, New York.

J. MICHAEL HENDERSON, F.R.C.S.
The Joseph B. Whitehead Department of Surgery, Emory University School of Medicine, Atlanta, Georgia.

J. BRUCE KNEELAND, M.D.
The New York Hospital-Cornell Medical Center, New York, New York.

R. J. R. KNOWLES, M.D.
The New York Hospital-Cornell Medical Center, New York, New York.

B. C. P. LEE, M.D.
The New York Hospital-Cornell Medical Center, New York, New York.

THOMAS D. ROHDE, M.S.
Department of Surgery, University of Minnesota, Minneapolis, Minnesota.

CARY L. STOWE, M.D.
Department of Surgery, Baylor College of Medicine and the Surgical Service of The Methodist Hospital, Houston, Texas.

W. DEAN WARREN, M.D.
The Joseph B. Whitehead Department of Surgery, Emory University School of Medicine, Atlanta, Georgia.

J. P. WHALEN, M.D.
The New York Hospital-Cornell Medical Center, New York, New York.

BRUCE G. WOLFF, M.D.
The Section of Colon & Rectal Surgery, Mayo Clinic, Rochester, Minnesota.

Table of Contents

Preservation of the Anorectum

BRUCE G. WOLFF, M.D.
AND
OLIVER H. BEAHRS, M.D.

The Section of Colon & Rectal Surgery, Mayo Clinic, Rochester, Minnesota

THE ANAL SPHINCTER is a complex and highly specialized muscular and neurologic phenomenon with a sophistication that has been appreciated for hundreds of years. Oddly enough, the research attention and physiologic mechanisms associated with the anus and anal canal have only recently begun to receive much import. The advent of procedures such as the ileal endorectal pull-through, as well as some devices such as the EEA stapler have more recently focused attention on proper reconstruction of the lower rectum and anal canal and the achieving of continence. Reevaluation of older techniques, such as the colo-anal operations, has been the biproduct of the desire to preserve the anus. As the population of elderly patients enlarges, rectal prolapse and the descending perineum syndrome, with or without accompanying incontinence, have become more prevalent and rectal excision with a permanent colostomy for these benign conditions seems more and more to be an excessive measure.

In discussing procedures that would preserve anal function, it is extremely important to bear in mind the determinants of continence. There are four principle regulating factors for continence and some preoperative assessment of these factors should be made, particularly in a situation in which one or more of these factors may be changed by the procedure contem-

0065-3411/84/0018-0001-0036-$04.00

plated. The four factors are (1) the anal sphincters, (2) the anorectal angulation, (3) the reservoir capacity of the rectum, and (4) the volume and consistency of the stools. An example of the disturbance of the interrelationship of these four factors would be the straight ileoanal endorectal pull-through *without* a reservoir, which generally was performed several years ago. Many patients did well with this straight anastomosis despite lacking a reservoir capacity of a neorectum. Many others, however, did not fare well and, in time, the reservoir was added to the operation. Many patients whose sphincter function was suboptimal found that lack of this reservoir was intolerable.

In discussing the anal sphincters we should remember that the anal canal itself frequently is divided into the anatomical anal canal and the surgical anal canal. In other words, the dentate line to the anal verge, or anatomical anal canal, is different from the surgical anal canal, which is the area between the puborectalis, well above the dentate line, to the anal verge. The length of the surgical anal canal is 3–4 cm and consists of the internal sphincter, which contains nerve endings that, through somewhat yet obscure mechanisms, can discriminate between gas, fluid, and solid in the anal canal. The internal sphincter also provides for a substantial part of the resting tone of the anal canal. The voluntary sphincters, consisting of the puborectalis, the superficial external sphincter, and the subcutaneous external sphincter, provide the major mechanism of continence. The entire sphincter mechanism is felt to function as a single unit, largely through the conjoined longitudinal muscle that sends fibers throughout the aforementioned other muscles, and is a continuation of the longitudinal muscle layer of the colon.

The anorectal angle (the angle formed between the anal canal and the lower rectum when viewed from a true lateral aspect, and in normal subjects is ≤ 90 degrees) is simply a radiographic delineation of the upper border of the anal canal formed by the levator muscles and, more specifically, by the puborectalis. The puborectalis is probably the most critical of all muscles for continence. If the subcutaneous and superficial external sphincters are cut, continence for solids, for liquids, and even for gas can be retained if the puborectalis sling is intact. This angle can be examined on a true lateral view of a defecating proctogram using either videotape or spot films. Loss of this angle provides a straight channel and, thus, a natural barrier to anal soiling is lost. However, many patients who have lost this angle can still retain continence if the external sphincters are intact and functioning. Patients with descending perineum syndrome and with rectal prolapse will have this angulation obliterated by severe dilatation and spreading of the fibers of the puborectalis.

The reservoir capacity of the rectum is another key factor in continence and any attempt at replacing the rectum should take this capacity into account. Finally, the volume and stool consistency is another interrelated factor with the optimum condition being semisoft, formed stool and the avoidance of watery diarrhea and very hard stools at the extremes.

In summary, preservation of the anal canal optimally includes voluntary control of defecation, the ability to distinguish the quality of rectal contents, and the ability to maintain nocturnal continence. We have yet to see a procedure in which the anorectum itself or all of its functions can be replaced, but progress is rapidly being made as the finer points of anorectal physiology are elucidated.

Benign Conditions

RECTAL PROLAPSE

One condition that can be reversed by a surgical approach with preservation or restoration of continence is rectal prolapse. In middle-aged and younger patients in whom the condition is not long-standing, elimination of the prolapsing segment of rectum or colon by any of the several techniques currently being used (anterior resection, modified Ripstein procedure, or Well's Ivalon® sponge procedure) will, in time, bring restoration of continence as the stretched anal sphincter fibers return to a normal configuration. However, if the prolapse is grade 3, and is long-standing, the stretch fibers frequently cannot respond or there has been neurologic damage. Occasionally, an indication of the status of the sphincter mechanism and pudendal nerve can be gained by performing preoperative anal manometry. Matheson and Keighley performed manometry in 63 patients with complete rectal prolapse or fecal incontinence, or both, and compared the results with the equal number of age- and sex-matched controls.[1] Maximum basal pressure or resting pressure and maximum squeeze pressure were measured before surgical treatment and four months and one year postoperatively. Patients with rectal prolapse alone had normal anal pressures, whereas patients with incontinence with or without prolapse had significantly lower resting and squeeze pressures than did the control subjects. While successful surgical treatment of prolapse or incontinence failed to produce a rise in anal canal pressures, continence was restored in most of these patients. With the addition of pelvic floor exercises and a reeducation process in teaching patients to squeeze, there was a significant rise in maximum squeeze pressure.

Keighley and Matheson also reported on a series of 56 patients treated for rectal prolapse and incontinence.[2] Of 32 patients with complete rectal prolapse, 25 had associated incontinence. The procedure performed for prolapse was the Ivalon® sponge technique with a partial wrapping of the mobilized rectum and rectopexy. Rectopexy was successful in treating rectal prolapse in all cases and only four of the patients with incontinence and prolapse remained incontinent after rectopexy alone. With the use of the postanal repair procedure, in which a plane is created posterior to the rectum between internal and external sphincters and the puborectalis fibers are brought together posterior to the rectum by interrupted sutures, the rectum is brought forward and the anorectal angle is reconstituted. Three of the four incontinent patients regained continence and the fourth has shown some improvement after postanal repair. Therefore, using a combination of these surgical treatment techniques, first dealing with the rectal prolapse and then, if necessary, with the weak pelvic floor, 45 of 48 patients who were initially incontinent were improved (4%) and 87% achieved complete control of defecation.

In addition to anal manometry, a defecating proctogram frequently can aid in the decision to perform a postanal repair after rectopexy or anterior resection if continence has not been restored. In most cases however, the posterior fixation of the rectum into the sacral hollow occurs by scarring or by the insertion of a foreign material. Suturing this material (Ivalon® or Teflon® mesh) to the rectum often will reconstitute the anorectal angle and improve continence by this simple measure alone.

The decision of which operation to perform for rectal prolapse is a controversial one. Beahrs and Theuerkauf reported a recurrence rate of only 3.7% out of 28 of anterior resection cases (and one death).[3] In this procedure, the rectum (except in the case of the first patient in which there was a recurrence) was mobilized to the level of the levator ani muscles. In a more recent review of 115 patients followed for more than three years, there was a rectal prolapse recurrence rate of 11%.[4]

The Ripstein procedure[5] has had a reported recurrence rate of 2.3%, from a sample of more than a thousand Ripstein procedures performed by 159 colon and rectum surgeons, that has not been duplicated by reports from the Lahey Clinic (recurrence rate of 7.5%) or the Cleveland Clinic (recurrence rate of 12.2%).[6] The Ivalon® sponge technique also has a low recurrence rate, but has problems associated with infection secondary to the sponge itself and the recurrence rate is somewhat higher than that reported with anterior resection or with the Ripstein procedure. In very-poor-risk elderly patients, an Altmeier procedure or rectosigmoidectomy can be performed with anal preservation. A parasacral approach also has been described using the York-Mason (Bevan) technique with posterior division of the anal sphincters without resection. Anterior approximation of the levator musculature and posterior fixation of the rectum are accomplished through this procedure.[7] The Thiersch wire procedure performed using an elastic material, such as a Silastic sheet, also has been reported.[8, 9]

RECTOVAGINAL FISTULA

In the irradiated rectum with a concomitant rectovaginal fistula there is another recent advancement. Bricker and Johnston[10] have reported the results of 21 operations for repair of rectovaginal fistula or stricture secondary to irradiation for pelvic cancer. The operations rely on the use of proximal nonirradiated colon with a normal blood supply and with an anastomosis made to the anterior rectal wall without mobilization of the rectal ampulla or by entering the presacral space. This is done either by an abdominal or a combined abdominoperineal approach. Eighteen of nineteen patients had a satisfactory to excellent functional result and one patient had a poor result. Two operations out of the 21 were total failures. most of these procedures were for reestablishment of continuity after a defunctionalizing colostomy that the authors say always should be performed.

In another study from the Cleveland Clinic by Lavery and associates[11] of 50 patients with radiation injury treated surgically, 41 had external diversions. Eleven had intestinal continuity restored, but diversion alone was not sufficient treatment in 11 patients. They concluded that diversion was the safest form of treatment for rectovaginal fistulas, rectal strictures, and proctitis that was unresponsive to medical therapy. They also noted that intestinal resection resulted in increased morbidity and mortality.

VILLOUS ADENOMA

Villous adenomas of the rectum frequently pose difficult problems for the surgeon and rarely are so extensive that abdominoperineal resection is required, however, up to 40% of these tumors may have a malignant component. In a series of 194 cases reported from the Mayo Clinic from 1950 to 1963,[12] 98% of these tumors were treated successfully with conservative means; that is, with electrocoagulation or excision. Examination of the surgical specimens from 11 patients treated by radical excision (mostly abdominoperineal resection) showed that conservative treatment would have been adequate because most of these lesions were confined to the mucosa.

Many of these smaller tumors can be prolapsed and removed by local transanal excision when located up to 12 cm from the anal verge. The mucosa in older patients is quite flexible and an endorectal local excision can be accomplished with suture reapproximation of the tissue as the lesion is excised. For more extensive circumferential villous tumors, a surgical method, in which the submucosal plane is developed to dissect the tumor off of the muscularis, is started. After circumferential excision of the tumor, the muscularis is plicated to allow the proximal mucosa to be brought down so that suturing to the dentate line can be performed.[13] This excision is done in much the same fashion as the mucosal proctectomy for an ileoanal procedure.

For favorable lesions, particularly located on the anterior aspect of the rectum, a York-Mason procedure may be performed.[14] With the patient in a jackknife position, complete division of the anal sphincters can be performed posteriorly, but this necessitates careful reapproximation of each muscle layer at the conclusion of the procedure. The exposure of the lower and middle rectum is excellent in this procedure. With meticulous reapproximation of the levators, the puborectalis, and the external and internal sphincters, complete continence and normal defecation are assured. This procedure was actually described first in 1917 by Dr. Arthur D. Bevan of Chicago, but the transsphincteric approach was only more recently popularized in Britain by York-Mason.[15] Knowledge of the anorectal musculature is essential for successful employment of this anal preservation procedure.

INFLAMMATORY BOWEL DISEASE

The patient with inflammatory bowel disease provides a myriad of choices for the surgeon. The need for surgery can be divided into two categories, emergency and elective surgery. The emergency indications are free perforation, massive hemorrhage, toxic megacolon, and fulminating colitis.[16] The elective indications for surgery in inflammatory bowel disease that arise from associated complications (particularly those of Crohn's disease) are failure to thrive in the teenage patient, stricture with partial obstruction, chronic abscess or fistula, and bleeding. Also important to consider are the chronic debilitation from the disease process and such extracolonic complications as pyoderma gangrenosum, periarteritis nodosa, and uveitis. An additional consideration is the malignant potential with ulcerative colitis and also the much-diminished, although real, potential in Crohn's disease. The opportunities and indications for rectal preservation in inflammatory bowel disease have come under close scrutiny in recent years and are still evolving. The increased use of specific studies of anorectal function in the future may play a key role in patient selection for anorectal preservation procedures.

CROHN'S DISEASE

It is known that patients with ileocolitis have a high incidence of recurrence in Crohn's disease. Indeed, the natural history of Crohn's disease is eventual recurrence, but the timing of the recurrence or extension is indeterminate. Of interest in this regard, is a study from the Cleveland Clinic[17] of 101 patients who had subtotal colectomy with rectal preservation; 58 of them eventually underwent either rectal excision or ileorectal anastomosis. The key question is, What is the fate of the rectum in patients who have anorectal Crohn's disease and, as a separate group, patients who have an ileorectostomy for Crohn's disease? In a recent follow-up (> 10 years) of 74 patients[18] with anorectal Crohn's disease, it was found that only 14 had had anorectal resection. However, if there was extensive proximal disease, the cumulative probability of retaining the rectum was 64% as opposed to 97% if the patient had no proximal disease. It was also noted that there was no significant lasting improvement with proximal resection of active anorectal Crohn's disease in this period of time. However, metronidazole, if tolerated for long periods of time, may produce healing or remission of anorectal Crohn's disease,[19] but this needs further evaluation. Alexander-Williams has promoted a conservative approach in surgery for fissures and fistulas in patients with anorectal Crohn's disease and has shown that over a period of 10 years in a group of 109 patients with anorectal Crohn's disease, only 10 required excision of the rectum and only 5 of these operations were for perianal disease. Moreover, in the vast majority, the fissures and fistulas had healed spontaneously or were asymptomatic.[20]

In patients with severe anorectal Crohn's disease, the process of completely diverting the fecal stream in the hope that, with the healing of the rectum, intestinal continuity would be restored has not generally been proved to be effective. McIlrath from the Mayo Clinic observed 13 patients who were treated in this fashion, four subsequently underwent proctocolectomy because of perianal complications and only two underwent subsequent reestablishment of intestinal continuity subsequent to resolution of anorectal Crohn's disease.[21] Diversion has also been found not to be of value by Korelitz.[22] He found that in 23 patients undergoing diversion the rectal segment became progressively inflamed and stricture was a prominent component. He noted that an early reanastomosis reversed these changes.

Ileorectal anastomosis frequently is employed in Crohn's disease in order to reestablish continuity after resection and to allow maintenance of continence even in a rectum that contains active Crohn's disease. In attempting to predict which patients would benefit from an ileorectal anastomosis, Keighley[23] preoperatively evaluated anal squeeze pressures and compliance by balloon distention in 53 patients who subsequently underwent ileorectal anastomosis. He found that anal squeeze pressure was of no benefit in predicting outcome, whereas the rectal compliance correlated well with an acceptable result. Buchmann and associates, in a review of the cumulative risks of reoperation of 105 patients with Crohn's disease and ileorectal anastomosis, found that half of these patients required reoperation within 20 years, although not all of them required proctectomy; fifty percent retained the rectum and had a satisfactory result.[24]

In the Mayo Clinic experience with intractable and complicated ileocolitis or Crohn's colitis patients who come to surgery, panproctocolectomy and ileostomy or an abdominal colectomy with a ileorectal anastomosis have been the only two common surgical choices. Farnell and associates,[25] in reviewing the cases of 80 patients with Crohn's colitis or ileocolitis who underwent an ileorectal anastomosis, found that 42 (61%) of the patients had an intact and functioning rectum after a mean follow-up of eight years. However, many of these patients were having 10 to 15 bowel movements per day with occasional incontinence. After employing certain objective criteria outlined in this chapter, viz., (1) more than eight bowel movements per day, (2) the need for systemic steroid use, (3) incontinence, and (4) poor general health, it was found that only 24 of 69 evaluable patients (35%) had a satisfactory result. In nearly 90% of these patients at the time of operation, the rectum was proctoscopically normal or only moderately diseased (19%). Operative mortality was 1.3% and there were no anastomotic leaks. Twenty-three (29%) eventually came to proctectomy and another 5% had a permanent ileostomy with the rectum in place. The operation was a frank failure in 27 (34%). Since the rectum is normal, or only moderately diseased, a diverting ileostomy or two-stage procedure is not generally performed. We feel that an ileorectal anastomosis is an excellent alternative (1) if the rectum is proctoscopically normal or minimally diseased, (2) if the anal sphincters are intact and there is minimal anorectal disease (no fissures or fistulas), (3) if the rectum is compliant as determined by barium study, (4) if anal sphincters function satisfactorily based on anal manometry, and (5) if there is enough small bowel to provide adequate nutritive absorptive surface.

ULCERATIVE COLITIS

It is in the group of young ulcerative colitis patients who come to surgery, and many do, that options have improved tremendously in the last 10 years. Prior to the early 1970s, proctocolectomy and a Brooke ileostomy was the standard choice for these patients, and this safe and effective operation is still the benchmark for comparison of all subsequent procedures.

Ileorectostomy, as reported by Aylett,[26] has become popular in Britain and in Australia and has received a strong following in the United States as well. It is usually a staged procedure with abdominal colectomy and ileorectostomy and a proximal diverting ileostomy that is closed at a later date. Proctectomy was required in only 7% of Aylett's series of more than 400 patients and 87% had a satisfactory result. However, almost 6% of these patients developed a carcinoma in the retained rectum.

In 1961–73 at the Mayo Clinic,[27] this procedure was performed in 63 patients with either absent or only mild rectal mucosal disease. The operative mortality was 3.2%. Diverting ileostomy was not routinely performed. The operative mortality was 3.2% and one patient developed a clinical leak requiring diverting ileostomy. There were 12 late deaths of which six were disease related. Of the 49 patients alive at follow-up, 22 (45%) had an unsatisfactory clinical result based on the criteria of (1) more than eight bowel movements per day, (2) need for systemic steroid use, (3) incontinence, and (4) poor general health. Fifteen patients underwent a proctectomy at a later time. Of the 33 patients left with an intact, functioning anastomosis, clinical results were considered unsatisfactory based on the above criteria in six patients. An earlier report from this Institution noted a 5.7% incidence of carcinoma of the rectum in 35 patients who had undergone ileorectostomy.[28]

The deficiencies of ileorectostomy in ulcerative colitis are the residual disease located in the rectum and the diminished, although concrete, risk of carcinoma in the rectal segment. The concept and role of dysplasia and rectal biopsy is still controversial and may well become moot in the future as newer procedures are applied. In addition, it must be remembered that, in any operation for colonic inflammatory disease, the distinction between chronic ulcerative colitis and Crohn's colitis is either impossible or a misdiagnosis in 10% of the cases.

In 1969, Kock[29] reported the experience with an ileal pouch serving as a reservoir for small bowel contents after proctocolectomy (Fig 1). Subsequent development of a "nipple valve" and subsequent modification have brought this procedure up to a more satisfactory and successful technique in which Kock was able to reduce his nipple revision rate to 26%, although Goligher has reported a failure rate of 40%.[30] In the series reported from the Mayo Clinic by Dozois et al.,[31] there were no surgical deaths in 299 patients on whom this procedure was performed. The pouch was excised in 10% of the first 149 of these patients and in only 3% of the second 150. The valve revision rate in the first 149 was 43%, whereas this had dropped to 22% in the second 150 patients. This result represents changes in techniques such as lengthening of the nipple valve and stapling of the nipple. Ninety-five percent of the patients reached a level of continence in which they did not have to wear an appliance, but in some of these patients this was achieved only after several operations. Seventy-five percent of the patients achieved complete continence. In a subsequent paper in which factors affecting revision rate after continent ileostomy were analyzed, Dozois and colleagues[32] noted that older patients were more prone to have potentially serious postoperative complications and to have multiple revisional procedures than younger patients. Also, patients with Crohn's disease and obese patients did not fare well with this procedure. The psychological state of the patient in his or her willingness to face revisional procedures and complications must also be taken into account.

Continence in an ileostomy also could be achieved through use of an enterostomal indwelling valve (Fig 2). This was developed and went through a trial first in dogs and then in humans with a conventional Brooke ileostomy.[33, 34] Although continence can be achieved in a straight ileostomy with this "continent ostomy valve," it has found wider usage in patients with a Kock pouch who have nipple valve reduction or in patients in whom a valveless ileal reservoir has been constructed specifically for use with this device.[35] In addition, candidates

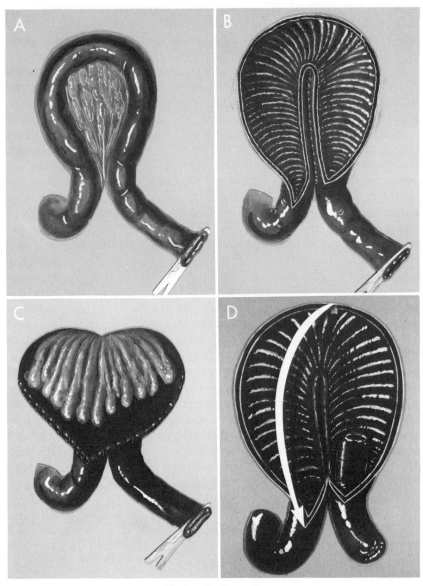

Fig 1.—Kock pouch.

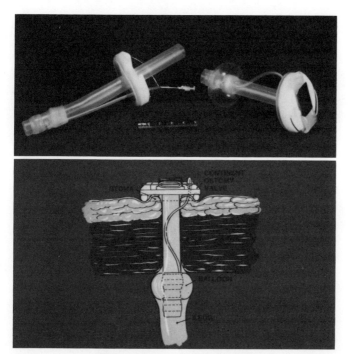

Fig 2.—Continent ostomy valve.

for this type of procedure are older patients and obese patients for whom a Kock ileostomy and, more specifically, conversion from a Brooke ileostomy is not feasible. This device is not recommended for use in patients with Crohn's disease.[36]

Recently, a procedure described by Parks[37] and Utsunomiya[38] and that we will refer to as the ileal pouch-anal anastomosis procedure has gained a great deal of enthusiasm (Fig 3). Experience with a straight endorectal ileoanal anastomosis without a pouch[39] has shown that a pouch, or some sort of rectal reservoir, can improve results in this type of procedure, which comes closest to restoration of normal anatomy with continence after total abdominal colectomy and mucosal proctectomy.[40] In a study by Heppell and colleagues,[41] the need for a pouch was clearly demonstrated as well as the effectiveness of preservation of the anal sphincter. The advantages of the procedure are obvious in that, in chronic ulcerative colitis and in familial polyposis, it removes all of the diseased mucosa,

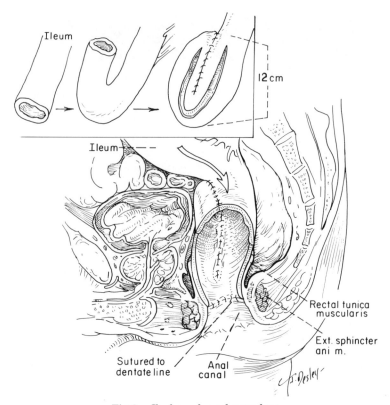

Fig 3.—Ileal pouch-anal procedure.

avoids a permanent abdominal stoma, retains continence through use of the anal sphincters, does not disturb innervation of the bladder and genitalia, and avoids a perineal wound. The only abnormality found on postoperative anal manometry is that the rectal inhibitory reflex is present in only roughly one fourth of the patients, but this does not seem to have a pronounced functional effect and needs to be investigated further.

A current surgical technique for this procedure is as follows. The anesthetized patient is positioned synchronously for a combined approach to the abdomen and perineum. The lower midline incision is made and a total abdominal colectomy is done. In approaching the rectum from above, the dissection is carried close onto the posterior wall of the rectum particularly to preserve the hypogastric plexus and the levator musculature. Indeed, the pelvic dissection itself is carried down very close to the rectal wall on all sides, although this dissection is more difficult. The terminal ileum is then mobilized along the ileocolic artery and superior mesenteric artery up to the level of the pancreas obtaining as much length as possible. Occasionally, it is necessary in performing a J-type pouch procedure to divide the ileocolic artery itself at some distance from the secondary arcade. However, blood flow through the secondary arcade is usually excellent and there are no ischemic problems with this maneuver. Transverse incisions in the mesentery also can provide additional length to the distal portion of the ileum. Pathologic examination of the abdominal colon has confirmed that the process is, indeed, chronic ulcerative colitis and not Crohn's disease. A J-type pouch is constructed using running absorbable sutures or the GIA stapler. It is important to close holes on both sides of the pouch when using the GIA stapler. The rectal mucosectomy is carried out with the use of two Gelpi self-retaining retractors that are placed at right angles to each other at the level of the dentate line. The mucosa is carefully dissected off of the internal sphincter; frequently, injection of a hyaluronidase, Lidocaine, and epinephrine solution can facilitate this dissection. This dissection is carried circumferentially above the level of the levators, approximately 6 cm above the dentate line. The stapled rectal stump is then delivered into the anal canal through a hole made in the posterior wall above the levators. The removal of the rectal stump and rectal mucosa is then accomplished much in the fashion that the rectum is removed in an abdominoperineal resection, that is, by following the mucosal edge around on the sides to the front, carefully preserving the internal sphincter. This dissection can be quite difficult if there is severe scarring in the submucosa and if lower rectal disease is severe. However, use of the aforementioned solution and judicious use of a needle-point cautery can facilitate preservation of some of the internal sphincter in this situation.

The completed reservoir is then introduced through the cuff of anal canal musculature and a 1 cm incision is made transversally in the pouch. A mucosa-to-anodermal anastomosis is then constructed with interrupted absorbable sutures. Two soft Hemovac catheters are placed into the pelvis and brought out

the lower quadrants and a temporary loop ileostomy is constructed. The protective ileostomy is taken down in 8 to 12
weeks after there is radiographic evidence that the pouch has
healed without leaks (Fig 4). Routine manometric studies with
compliance are now being performed on these patients in an
attempt to avoid a poor result due to a noncompliant pouch or
anal sphincter dysfunction.

In eight patients in our series, a temporary ileostomy was
not performed and this worked well in seven patients, but
proved suboptimal in one patient with minimal rectal disease
and chronic ulcerative colitis. We feel that a temporary loop
ileostomy should always be done except in patients with
chronic ulcerative colitis who have no discernible rectal mucosal disease and are not on steroids. This is also, we feel, an
acceptable maneuver in patients with familial polyposis, although the numbers are small and this aspect of the procedure
needs further study.

From January 1978 to June 1983, 236 adult patients have
undergone abdominal colectomy, mucosal proctectomy, and ileoanal anastomosis at Mayo Clinic-affiliated hospitals.[42] Fifty
patients had the straight ileoanal anastomosis and, as has been
mentioned before,[43] indicated that a reservoir would improve

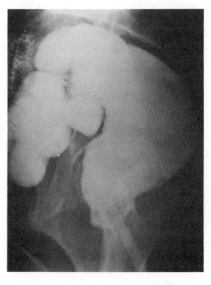

Fig 4.—"Pouchogram" showing a
capacious, well-healed ileal-anal pouch

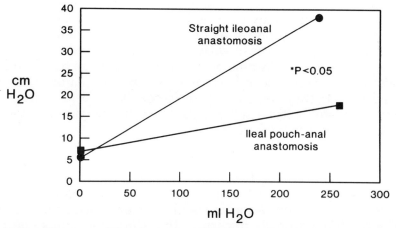

Fig 5.—Comparison of compliance of straight ileoanal procedure with ileal pouch-anal procedure.

the results of the procedure (Fig 5). The next 188 patients had the ileal pouch-anal procedure, 183 having a J-pouch and 5 having an S-pouch procedure. One hundred seventy-seven patients had chronic ulcerative colitis and 11 had polyposis. Intestinal continuity has been restored in 163 patients who are available for follow-up. There was no operative mortality in these patients, which has also been true for the Kock continent ileostomy patients. There have been 10 failures (5.3%) due to misdiagnosed Crohn's disease, intractable diarrhea, or pelvic sepsis. Pelvic sepsis occurred in 11% of these patients, but only 6.4% underwent laparotomy for this problem. The pouch has been excised in five patients (2.7%). Anastomotic strictures have occurred in 13.6% and bowel obstruction necessitating laparotomy in 7% after colectomy and in 2% after ileostomy closure. There are no cases of impotence, although there is a 9% incidence of retrograde ejaculation. Pouchitis occurred in 8.1% of these patients. All of these patients evacuate the pouch spontaneously and 95% of the patients prefer the ileal pouch-anal functional result to the ileostomy that they had for three months. The mean stools per day are 5.6 with 1.2 mean stools at night. Major leakage, defined as a patient's need to wear more than one pad per day, has been seen in 2.6% of the patients during the day. In an interval from 9 months to 18 months after ileostomy closure, it has been found that incontinence tended to improve, as did perineal irritation. Discrimination has also improved with time, and the need for medication has decreased. In nine patients older than age 50, in whom this procedure has been performed, the result has not been as good in that they have more stools per day and continence is less complete. It has also been observed that polyposis patients tend to have a better result.

In preoperative discussion of the options in patients with chronic ulcerative colitis, the advantages and disadvantages of proctocolectomy with Brooke ileostomy, ileorectostomy, Kock pouch, and pouch with the continent ostomy valve and the ileal pouch-anal anastomosis are carefully reviewed with the patient (Fig 6). It is extremely important that the patient make an intelligent decision on the type of operation to have, as well as to know all of the complications that may occur in each procedure, such as the high morbidity rate with the ileal pouch-anal procedure, as well as which operations have a good functional result. Also taken into consideration is the fact that there are no long-term results available and there may be long-term problems that may emerge with a newer procedure, such as the ileal pouch-anal anastomosis. However, we have been encouraged by generally excellent results of this procedure and patient satisfaction despite the significant risks of complications with it.

POLYPOSIS

Over the last 10 years there has been much controversy over the fate of the rectum in patients with familial polyposis syndromes (Fig 7). The conflict was perhaps sparked in 1971 by Adson and colleagues[44] who reported a very high incidence of rectal carcinoma in patients who had lengthy follow-up after ileosigmoidostomy or ileorectostomy. Several authors then reported series in which the incidence of carcinoma of the rectum in polyposis patients after ileorectostomy was not nearly as elevated.[45-49] In 1980, Adson and colleagues[50] reevaluated progress for the same group of patients and attempted to determine which factors might predispose a patient to carcinoma of the

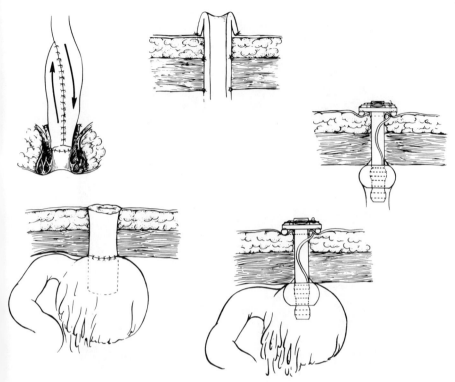

Fig 6.—Surgical alternatives in a patient with chronic ulcerative colitis.

rectum and which groups might represent a lesser risk of rectal carcinoma. Furthermore, in a recent elegant review of this topic,[51] a complete statement of the problem and associated disagreements is made. There is concensus that untreated patients with familial polyposis will develop colonic or rectal cancer if the bowel so predisposed is not removed; patients with colonic polyposis who have no rectal polyps are satisfactorily treated by colectomy and ileorectostomy. Removal of the colon proximal to the rectum seems to reduce the incidence or delay the appearance of rectal carcinoma in some patients.

There is disagreement about the appropriate level of ileorectal anastomosis and how much protection a lower rectal anastomosis would afford, about the effectiveness of fulguration of polyps in the rectal segment after ileorectostomy, about the

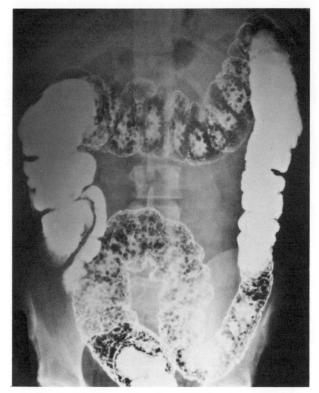

Fig 7.—Florid manifestation of Gardner's syndrome.

timing in operations in which the rectum is preserved by ileorectostomy, and about the correlations in the incidence of rectal
carcinoma with age, sex, number of colonic or rectal polyps,
family history, prior colonic cancer, and anastomotic level.

For years the only surgical alternatives in patients with polyposis was proctocolectomy and Brooke ileostomy, or ileorectostomy. There is now a third alternative, the ileal pouch-anal
procedure, which, if proved clinically successful, will make the
discussion over the two older alternatives moot. However, from
the studies of Adson,[52, 53] it seems that patients with less than
20 polyps in the rectal segment, male patients, and patients
who have no concomitant or previous colonic malignancy are at
a reduced risk for rectal carcinoma from ileorectostomy. However, the goal of the surgeon in this disorder should be to re-

move *any* risk of rectal malignancy, and the ileal pouch-anal procedure may well provide that opportunity. At the present time, in younger patients with familial polyposis who have roughly 20 polyps or less in the rectum, we perform a near-total abdominal colectomy with an ileosigmoidostomy, ideally located at about 15 cm providing an anastomosis within the peritoneal cavity that is serosally lined and that is performed without rectal mobilization. This protects the hypogastric plexus and, thus, sexual and bladder function, and allows for an easier dissection when the patient returns for ileoanal pouch-anal procedure at a later date. These patients are followed very closely and rectal polyps are destroyed as they are encountered. Then, at an age of 25 to 30 years, an ileal pouch-anal procedure can be performed with elimination of the remaining rectal mucosa at risk. Obviously we would proceed with a mucosal proctectomy at the first operation and perform the ileal pouch-anal procedure in older patients or in patients whose rectums are carpeted with polyps. These are only rough guidelines and individual cases must be viewed afresh from a point encompassing proctocolectomy with ileostomy, Kock pouch, ileorectostomy, and ileal pouch-anal procedures.

Malignant Disease

Rectal preservation or preservation of anal function also has undergone an evolutionary process over the past two decades. Undoubtedly, many abdominoperineal resections have been performed for malignant disease in which a sphincter-preserving procedure might have been done without increase in the risk of recurrence or jeopardizing the chance for a cure. This has been very aptly stated in the following quote:

The avoidance of a colostomy when indicated may jeopardize the patient's chance of cure and this is an unfortunate mistake in surgical judgement. Equally tragic is the sacrifice of the patient's anal sphincter mechanism and all semblance of normality without increasing his chance of survival.[54]

ANAL TUMORS

Malignant anal tumors are rare and the average surgeon will encounter, perhaps, only one or two in the course of a long and busy practice. They comprise only from 1% to 4% of colon and anorectal malignancies.[55, 56] In a review of anal cancer from the Mayo Clinic in 1976 by Beahrs and Wilson,[57] the following distribution of tumors was found: squamous cell carcinoma (55%), basaloid carcinoma (31%), Paget's disease (4%), melanoma (3.5%), basal cell carcinoma (3.5%), and adenocarcinoma (3.5%) (Fig 8). Other tumors found in this series included lymphosarcoma, leiomyosarcoma, rhabdomyosarcoma, hemangiopericytoma, plasmacytoma, and endothelioma. Many of these tumors are amenable, because of low grade or small size, to local excision.

SQUAMOUS CELL CARCINOMA/BASALOID CARCINOMA

Squamous cell carcinoma and basaloid carcinoma occur more commonly in women during the fifth and sixth decades. Major presenting symptoms are likely to be bleeding, pain, or an anal mass [58–60]; squamous cell carcinoma is likely to be associated with pruritus ani.[61] Basaloid carcinoma (transitional carcinoma, cloacogenic carcinoma) is considered by some authors[62] to be a nonkeratinizing squamous carcinoma behaviorally resembling an adenocarcinoma of the rectum. The hallmark of anal tumors is induration on examination. A lesion presenting in this fashion should be biopsied.

Squamous carcinoma that is superficial and low grade (that is, less than 2 cm in diameter) can be treated with wide local

Fig 8.—Areas of origin of anal tumors.

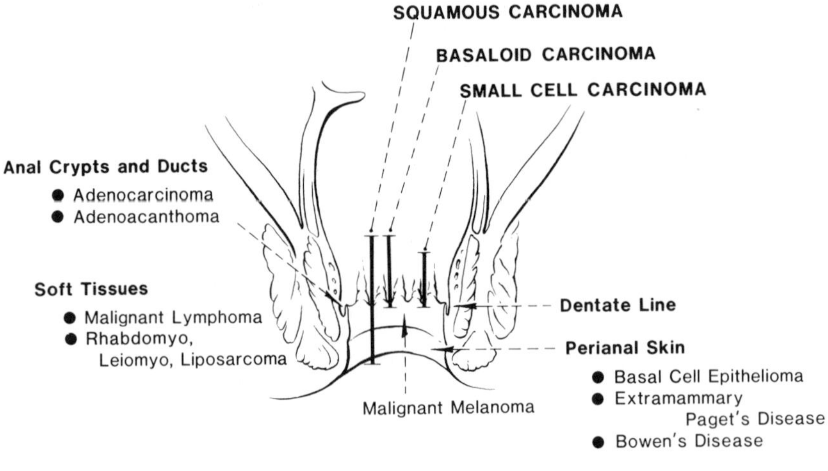

SQUAMOUS CARCINOMA

BASALOID CARCINOMA

SMALL CELL CARCINOMA

Anal Crypts and Ducts
● Adenocarcinoma
● Adenoacanthoma

Soft Tissues
● Malignant Lymphoma
● Rhabdomyo,
 Leiomyo, Liposarcoma

Dentate Line

Perianal Skin
● Basal Cell Epithelioma
● Extramammary
 Paget's Disease
● Bowen's Disease

Malignant Melanoma

excision. Recently, tumors larger than this have been biopsied and treated with a combination of mitomycin C, 5-fluorouracil, and radiation, resulting in anorectal preservation and complete disappearance of the tumor.[63][64] A multicenter prospective randomized trial is needed to obtain sufficient numbers to compare chemotherapy and radiation vs. surgical treatment in this tumor. However, in a recent report of a fairly large series of patients, 12 patients with stage A disease and tumors less than 2 cm in diameter had a 100% five-year survival, although one had a recurrence necessitating abdominoperineal excision.[65] Five of seven stage B patients had a local excision and four of the seven survived five years. Five-year survival for stage A patients, who underwent abdominoperineal resection (6 patients), was 83% and for stage B (76 patients), it was 74%. Most recurrences in this series were local rather than distant, which is somewhat different from the usual pattern seen in adenocarcinoma of the rectum.

The best proved treatment for larger invasive squamous cell carcinomas or basaloid carcinomas of the perianal area or anal canal is abdominoperineal excision. However, the combined radiation/chemotherapy approach may alter this approach in the future.

MELANOMAS

The anal canal is the third most common site for primary melanoma, although less than 1% of all melanomas arise in that area.[66] Thirty-seven cases of this rare tumor recently were analyzed.[67] Most of the tumors were larger than 2 cm. Despite wide local excision in the smaller tumors and abdominoperineal excision, only three patients survived for more than five years and none of the patients treated by abdominoperineal excision survived five years. There is a recent report in which a 50% five-year survival was achieved in six patients treated with a very radical surgery involving a posterior pelvic exenteration with incontinuity groin and pelvic nodal dissections.[68] Since abdominoperineal resection has not been shown to improve survival in these patients, perhaps local excision with anorectal preservation is a reasonable course in patients with larger tumors who are at considerable risk for recurrence in this highly fatal disease.

Other anal tumors and conditions in which local, rather than rectal, excision is the treatment of choice are basal cell carcinoma, Bowen's disease, perianal Paget's disease, and Buschke-Lowenstein tumor.[69]

RECTAL TUMORS

Another tumor which is very rare, but is occasionally seen, is a rectal lymphoma. This is a tumor in which rectal preservation is appropriate in most cases. Sixty-one such cases seen between 1950–77 recently have been reviewed at our institution.[70] Diagnosis was confirmed by mucosal biopsy on proctoscopy in 75% of the cases. Almost all of these patients were treated with radiation therapy and usually with complete resolution of the rectal lesions. The overall five-year survival rate was 20%. Those patients who had a localized process of the rectum had almost a 50% survival rate. Patients who had disease spread apart from the rectum had a lower survival rate. These patients died of widespread disease, complications of malnutrition, infection, or bleeding. The rectal involvement rarely produced a life-threatening situation.

RECTAL ADENOCARCINOMA

In patients with small polypoid rectal adenocarcinomas that are not deeply invasive, two alternatives to major resection with anorectal preservation are possible. One is intracavitary radiation as described by Papillon from Lyon, France. Through a process of strict selection in cases in 133 patients who were followed for more than five years, he reported a five-year survival rate of 78%.[71] An intracavitary radiation dose is given every two or three weeks and a total dose to the tumor varies between 9,000 and 12,500 rad over seven to eight weeks. There are surprisingly few complications with this technique. However, the lesions selected must be well-differentiated, they must be mobile with no penetration or fixation, they must be no larger than 5 cm in diameter, they must be located within 10 cm of the anal verge, and there should be no palpable lymphadenopathy.

A second method for preservation of anal function in rectal adenocarcinoma is electrocoagulation. In a series reported by

Salvatti and Rubin,[72] this procedure is performed with the patient in the lithotomy position under a light general anesthetic; extensive electrocoagulation requires an hour or more. All charred tumor is removed by biopsy forceps and the process is repeated. Several operative procedures may be necessary to remove the tumor. This procedure is particularly applicable in villous adenoma with superficial adenocarcinomas of the rectum. If hard lymphadenopathy occurs, palpable through the rectal wall next to the electrocoagulated area, this is an indication for abdominoperineal resection. The indication for electrocoagulation in good-risk patients is an adenocarcinoma within 7½ cm of the anal verge that occupies less than one-half the circumference of the rectum. The ideal lesion, again, is movable with no deep penetration or fixation. This technique has been used in poor-risk patients and the overall survival rate for 70 patients thus treated over a 13-year period was 49%. Seventeen of these patients required surgical resection and their survival was 41%. Hemorrhage is a prominent complication of this procedure and perforation occurred in two patients. It must be pointed out that the survival rate for Dukes A and B lesions should be better than 49%, so great care must be used in applying electrocoagulation in any patient for whom abdominoperineal resection would be curative.

Since Miles described the abdominoperineal procedure in 1908, this has been the procedure of choice for all resectable carcinomas of the rectum whether they occurred in the mid, upper, or lower parts of the rectum. For purposes of discussion the low rectum will be considered as representing that portion from 0 to 5 cm above the dentate line. The midrectum is described as 6 through 9 cm above the dentate line and the upper rectum as from 10 to 14 cm above the dentate line. Anterior resection preserving normal anorectal function was believed to have first been performed by Reybard in 1843.[73] Nicollet in 1903 reported a mortality rate from 30% to 50% with this procedure. He, therefore, explored the possibilities of an exteriorization technique and reduced his mortality rate to 12%. For the next 30 to 40 years, surgical treatment for cancer of the sigmoid and upper rectum consisted of a choice between exteriorization or abdominoperineal resection. In the 1940s the anterior resection, which had fallen into disrepute, again became generally accepted with the realization that rectal carcinoma did not spread distally on a routine basis as previously was thought. There is today very little disagreement that the surgical procedure of choice for carcinomas located in the lower one third of the rectum (from 0 to 5 cm) is the combined abdominoperineal resection; for carcinomas in the upper one third of the rectum (above 9 cm), anterior resection is clearly the procedure of choice. Controversy exists over carcinomas of the middle one third of the rectum that are located from 5 to 10 cm. Many surgeons favor low anterior resection for these lesions and others would perform a coloanal procedure (pull-through) or an abdominosacral type procedure as performed by Localio.[78]

The mortality rate for abdominoperineal resection today is less than 5% and the five-year survival rate is 50%. This, of course, is the standard to which local excision or a low anterior resection must be compared. Theoretically, out of 100 patients who have rectal carcinoma, 75 will have Dukes A and B lesions and will not benefit from an abdominoperineal resection. Of the remaining 25 patients with Dukes C lesions, approximately five will have hepatic metastasis at the time of surgery and, of the remaining 20 patients with Dukes C, one-half will be cured of their cancer by this procedure, at least, in theory. Since there is some mortality associated with the procedure, we can conclude that only five out of 100 patients would benefit from this procedure. The problem is in how to select the five who would benefit or would concomitantly benefit from low anterior resection or local excision.

In a series of anterior resections of 1,766 favorable lesions reported by Vandertoll and Beahrs,[74] the five-year survival rate for 1,741 patients who were followed up was 56%. The operative mortality rate in this series of patients was 4.2%. The pelvic recurrence rate for this series of patients was 11.5%, and 82% of these recurrences developed within three years. Of these patients, who had recurrent disease, two-thirds had a margin of normal bowel distal to the tumor in the excised specimen that was 3 cm or less. It seems reasonable to assume that some of these patients would have survived had a more radical abdominoperineal resection been done, but the fact remains that 56% of these patients were alive with normal bowel function five years after their procedure.

In deciding to perform low anterior resection, the following factors should be borne in mind. The resection should be an adequate cancer resection, including 3–5 cm of normal bowel below the lesion, and the use of careful technique with gentle handling of the tissues is important in this area where blood supply to the anastomosis plays a key role. The ends of the open bowel should be cleansed with irrigating agents, such as alcohol or Merthiolate. Drainage of the pelvis should be optimum with suction catheters. If there is doubt as to the adequacy of the anastomosis either on proctoscopy with air insufflation, while the abdomen is open and with the anastomosis covered by saline irrigation, or by inspection, a temporary colostomy should be performed. The decision as to whether a one- or a two-layer anastomosis is done is largely preferential, since in a 1977 report[75] there was only a slightly greater incidence of dehiscence after a one-layer technique of anastomosis for both anterior and low anterior resections. High-grade, bulky lesions should be treated by abdominoperineal resection. Abdominal transsacral resections and low anterior resections, as described by D'Allaines,[76] have the disadvantages of anastomotic leaks and recurrences; however, recently, the use of adjuvant radiation therapy has been shown to be effective in reducing pelvic or local recurrence.[77, 78] Vascular isolation of the tumor with a no-touch technique does not seem as important, when compared with survival, as the extent of resection.[79]

In a series of 400 patients with anterior resections for carcinoma of the rectum,[80] one-third of them being in the low anterior area, there was a 40% overall rate of complication. The overall leak rate was 5% and the leakage rate for lesions resected within 10 cm of the dentate line was 9%. This leakage rate was a clinical rate and, as has been reported by Goligher and colleagues,[81] almost 69% of patients in his series who underwent low anterior resection had a radiographically demonstrated leak; 51% who had a high anterior resection had a similar radiographic leak rate. It must also be noted that 57% of the patients who had leaks were managed satisfactorily without colostomy and that successful nonoperative management was possible, probably because suction pelvic drains were already in place. Dead space about the anastomosis in a low anterior resection, which limits contact with viable tissue that could adhere to seal off or even revascularize ischemic intestine, might well be a major cause of leakage. These authors have recommended a pedicle graft of viable omentum to be used to fill the dead space around the low anastomosis. They have demonstrated the reduction in leakage rate experimentally in dogs.[82]

Fecal incontinence in this series was no more likely to occur in patients who had low anterior resections than in those who had more proximal resections in a study by Akawari and Kelly.[83] Indeed, even though diarrhea was a significant postoperative problem in patients who underwent low anterior resection, in time adaptation seems to take place, with resolution of the symptoms even in very low anastomosis. In a paper from Japan,[84] 15 of 16 patients who underwent low anterior resection and who had frequent bowel movements and occasional soiling less than six months after their operation had complete resolution of those symptoms after six months. These authors demonstrated that there was close correlation between control of bowel movements and rectal compliance, but not between the resting pressure in the anal canal or the rectal inhibitory reflex.

The advent of the EEA stapling instrument undoubtedly has facilitated the construction of an anastomosis in low anterior resections. In 70 patients in a prospective randomized study, Beart and Kelly[85] showed that there was no difference in postoperative complications, including leak rate, between the traditional hand-sewn technique and the staple technique in situations where either can be used. The percentage of patients in their study who had the stapling device used to construct an anastomosis, rather than excision of the rectum, was 12%. These findings were confirmed by similar leak rates between the two techniques in a recent study reported by Brennan and colleagues.[86] A group from Sweden[87] has shown that, if a protective colostomy was done routinely, stenosis ensued. This was demonstrated in nine of 25 patients, compared with stenosis noted in only two out of 25 patients in the noncolostomy group. Therefore, they advised that routine protective colostomy should not be used in low anterior resection with the EEA stapling device.

However, the long-term results with the stapler in low anterior resection is just emerging. In a recent update by Beart and colleagues,[88] 190 patients with carcinoma in the midrectum who were similar in every other respect had a 29% incidence of local recurrence in the staple group as opposed to a 10% incidence in the nonstaple group. The reason for this is obscure, although it may be related to sample size or to the blood supply and reduced inflammation around the anastomosis, which has been thought to be present in EEA stapled cases.[89] Another thought is that stapled anastomoses are done in patients with tumors more likely to recur (narrow pelvis).

Some surgeons still prefer to use the abdominal endorectal resection or pull-through procedure rather than a low anterior resection.[90, 91] This procedure can be useful occasionally for a patient who has a small lesion in an extremely narrow pelvis or for a nonmalignant rectovaginal fistula repair; however, significant complications with this procedure have been reported, mainly pelvic sepsis[92] in 10% to 20% of the patients and sloughing of a portion of the colon in the pelvis. In addition, incontinence[93] has been noted to be a problem having been described as severe in 23% of the patients and minor in another 48%. Parks,[94] however, recently has reported 76 patients who between 1973–80 underwent rectal resection and restoration of bowel continuity by an anastomosis between the colon and the anal canal. Only two patients developed colonic necrosis and anastomotic breakdown and developed, as a consequence, pelvic sepsis. Sixty-nine of the seventy patients who could be assessed either had completely normal bowel function or only minor deficiencies. Six patients developed recurrent pelvic tumor and five-year survival rates were comparable to patients undergoing abdominoperineal resection.

Parks denudes the rectal stump of mucosa before performing the pull-through and coloanal anastomosis with 3–0 polyglycolic acid. In addition, he performs a temporary transverse loop colostomy. In 29 patients, the tumor was located between 4 and 8 cm from the anal margin and in 36 patients, the tumor was located between 8 and 12 cm; the remainder were above 12 cm. The mean distance of normal margin below the level of the tumor was 2.9 cm. The defunctioning colostomy, he notes, will not prevent colonic necrosis or anastomotic leakage, but frequently obviates the development of an extensive pelvic abscess. Parks and Lean[95] manometrically studied 12 patients who had a coloanal anastomosis and found that the rectum was not essential for discrimination, particularly of impending colonic evacuation, or for a rectal inhibitory reflex to be present.

In our own institution, Beart[96] has performed 10 such procedures for rectal carcinoma for the following indications: small tumors in which a pursestring suture placement for stapling or hand-sewn anastomosis was very difficult, and in a patient with a benign, radiation-induced, rectovaginal fistula.

The emergence and standardization of new diagnostic procedures, such as anal manometry with compliance, rectal electromyelography, the saline infusion test for incontinence, and the defecating proctogram are allowing more objective and critical assessment of diseased states in an anorectal function. These are particularly applicable in patients with benign disease of the lower colon and rectum and procedures for correcting detected abnormalities, such as the postanal repair for the descending perineum syndrome, have come forth. Perhaps, in the future, computerized tomography and magnetic resonance scans will enable better and more complete preoperative planning in rectal carcinoma, even to the point of determining which patients are good candidates for a local excision of their rectal carcinoma, rather than a complete rectal excision. Although vast improvement has occurred with the technique of irrigating the colostomy and in colostomy appliances, preservation of the normal channel for rectal evacuation and the indications and patient selection for this preservation are an absolute goal, and events of interest in this field are coming rapidly.

REFERENCES

1. Matheson D.M., Keighley M.R.B.: Manometric evaluation of rectal prolapse and fecal incontinence. *Gut* 22:126, 1981.
2 Keighley M.R.B., Matheson D.M.: Results of treatment for rectal prolapse and fecal incontinence. *Dis. Colon Rectum* 24:449, 1981.
3. Theuerkauf F.J., Jr., Beahrs O.H., Hill J.R.: Rectal prolapse: causation and surgical treatment. *Ann. Surg.* 171:819, 1970.
4. Schlinkert R., Wolff B.G., Pemberton J.H., et al.: Anterior resection for rectal prolapse. Presented at the American Society of Colon and Rectal Surgeons Convention, New Orleans, May 6–10, 1984.
5. Gordon P.H., Hoexter B.: Complications of Ripstein procedure. *Dis. Colon Rectum* 21:277, 1978.
6. Launer D.P., Fazio V.W., Weakly F.L., et al.: The Ripstein procedure: a 16-year experience. *Dis. Colon Rectum* 25:41, 1982.
7. Woods J.H., DeCosse J.J.: A parasacral approach to rectal prolapse. Arch Surg. 3:914, 1976.

8. Labow S., Rubin R.J., Hoexter B., et al.: Perineal repair of rectal procidentia with an elastic fabric sling. *Dis. Colon Rectum* 23:467, 1980.
9. Thorlakson R.H.: A modification of the Thiersch procedure for rectal prolapse using polyester tape. *Dis. Colon Rectum* 25:57, 1982.
10. Bricker E.M., Johnston W.D., Patwardhan R.V.: Repair of post irradiation damage to colorectum: a progress report. *Ann. Surg.* 193:555, 1981.
11. Anseline E.F., Lavery I.C., Fazio V.W., et al.: Radiation of the rectum: evaluation of surgical treatment. *Ann. Surg.* 194:716, 1981.
12. Ramariz R.F., Culp C.E., Jackman R.J., et al.: Villous tumors of the lower part of the large bowel. *JAMA* 194:863, 1965.
13. Gross W., Rubin R.J., Salvatti E.P., et al.: The method of management of a circumferential villous tumor of the rectum. *Dis. Colon Rectum* 24:151, 1981.
14. York-Mason A.: Surgical access to the rectum—a transsphincteric exposure. *Proc. R. Soc. Med.* 63:91, 1970.
15. Criado F.J., Wilson T.H.: Posterior transsphincteric approach for surgery of the rectum: the Bevan operation. *Dis. Colon Rectum* 24:145, 1981.
16. Beart R.W., Jr., McIlrath D.C., Kelly K.A., et al.: Surgical management of inflammatory bowel disease. *Curr. Prob. Surg.* 17:10, 1980.
17. Lock M.R., Fazio V.W., Farmer R.G., et al.: Proximal recurrence in the fate of the rectum following excisional surgery for Crohn's disease of the large bowel. *Surgery* 194–754:60, 1981.
18. Wolff B.G.: Unpublished data, 1983.
19. Bernstein L.H., Frank M.S., Brant L.J., et al.: Healing of perineal Crohn's disease with metronidazole. *Gastroenterol.* 79:357, 1980.
20. Buchmann P., Keighley M.R.B., Allan R.N., et al.: Natural history of perianal Crohn's disease: a 10-year follow-up; a plea for conservatism. *Am. J. Surg.* 140:642, 1980.
21. McIlrath D.C.: Diverting ileostomy or colostomy in the management of Crohn's disease of the colon. *Arch Surg.* 103:308, 1971.
22. Korelitz B.I.: Diversion of fecal stream in patients with Crohn's said not to be of long-term benefit. *Int. Med. News* 16:2, 1982.
23. Keighley M.R.G., Buchmann P., Lee J.R.: Assessment of anorectal function in selection of patients for ileorectal anastomosis in Crohn's colitis. *Gut* 23:102, 1982.
24. Buchmann P., Weteiman I.T., Keighley M.R.B., et al.: Prognosis of ileorectal anastomosis in Crohn's disease. *Br. J. Surg.* 68:7, 1981.
25. Farnell M.B., vanHeerden J.A., Beart R.W., Jr., et al.: Rectal preservation in nonspecific inflammatory diseases of the colon and rectum. *Ann. Surg.* 192:249, 1980.
26. Aylett F.O.: Rectal conservation in surgical treatment of ulcerative colitis. *Arch. Fr. Mal. Appl. Dig.* 63:585, 1974.
27. Farnell M.B., vanHeerden J.A., Beart R.W., Jr., et al.: Rectal preservation in nonspecific inflammatory disease of the colon. *Ann. Surg.* 192:249, 1980.
28. Adson M.A., Kauferman A.M., Farrow G.M.: Ileorectostomy for ulcerative colitis disease of the colon. *Arch. Surg.* 104:424, 1972.
29. Kock N.G.: Intra-abdominal "reservoir" in patients with permanent ile-

ostomy: preliminary observations on a procedure resulting in fecal "continence" in five ileostomy patients. *Arch. Surg.* 99:229, 1969.

30. Goligher J.C.: The quest for continence in the surgical treatment of ulcerative colitis. *Adv. Surg.* 14:53, 1980.

31. Dozois R.R., Kelly K.A., Beart R.W., Jr., et al.: Improved results with continence ileostomy. *Ann. Surg.* 192:319, 1980.

32. Dozois R.R., Kelly K.A., Ilstrup D., et al.: Factors effecting revision rate after continent ileostomy. *Arch. Surg.* 116:610, 1981.

33. Pemberton J.H., Kelly K.A., Phillips S.F.: Achieving ileostomy continence with an indwelling stomal device. *Surgery* 90:336, 1981.

34. Pemberton J.H., vanHeerden J.A., Beart R.W., Jr., et al.: A continent ileostomy device. *Ann. Surg.* 197:618–26, 1983.

35. Pemberton J.H., Kelly K.A., Beart R.W., Jr.: Achieving ileostomy continence with a prestomal ileal pouch in a stomal occlusive device. *Surgery* 94:72, 1983.

36. Pemberton J.H., Dozois R.R.: Continent ileostomy. *Problems in General Surgery—New Approaches to Old Problems.* 1:27–38, 1984.

37. Parks A., Nicholls R., Belliveau P.: Proctocolectomy with ileal reservoir and anal anastomosis. *Br. J. Surg.* 67:533, 1980.

38. Utsunomyia J., Iwama T., Imajo M., et al.: Total colectomy, mucosal proctectomy, and ileoanal anastomosis. *Dis. Colon Rectum* 23:459, 1980.

39. Beart R.W., Jr., Dozois R.R., Kelly K.A.: Ileoanal anastomosis in the adult. *Surg. Gynecol. Obstet.* 154:826, 1982.

40. Taylor B.M., Cranley B., Kelly K.A., et al.: A clinicophysiological comparison of ileal pouchanal and straight ileoanal anastomosis. *Ann. Surg.* 198:462, 1983.

41. Heppell J., Kelly K.A., Phillips S.F., et al.: Physiologic aspects of continence after colectomy, mucosal proctectomy, and endorectal ileoanal anastomosis.

42. Metcalf A.M., Dozois R.R., Wolff B.G., et al.: Ileal Pouch-Anal Results. Presented at the American Society of Colon and Rectal Surgeons Convention, New Orleans, May 6–10, 1984.

43. Beart R.W., Jr., Dozois R.R., Kelly K.A.: Ileoanal anastomosis in the adult. *Surg. Gynecol. Obstet.* 184:826, 1982.

44. Moertel C.G., Hill J.R., Adson M.A.: Management of multiple polyposis of the large bowel. *Cancer* 28:160, 1971.

45. Gingold B.S., Jagelman D., Turnbull R.B.: Surgical managment of familial polyposis and Gardner's syndrome. *Am. J. Surg.* 37:54, 1979.

46. Gingold B.S., Jagelman D.: Sparing the rectum with familial polyposis: causes for failure. *Surgery* 89:314, 1981.

47. Schaupp W.C., Volpe P.A.: Management of diffuse colonic polyposis. *Am. J. Surg.* 124:218, 1972.

48. Harvey J.C., Quan S.H., Stearns M.W.: Management of familial polyposis with preservation of the rectum. *Surgery* 84:476, 1978.

49. Alm T.: Surgical treatment of hereditary adenomatosis of the colon and rectum in Sweden during the last 20 years. *Acta. Chir. Scand.* 141:228, 1975.

50. Bess M.A., Adson M.A., Elveback L.R., et al.: Rectal cancer following colectomy for polyposis. *Arch. Surg.* 115:460, 1980.

51. Adson M.A., Farnell M.B.: Ileorectostomy: clinical results and current role, in Dozois R.R. (ed.): *Alternatives to Conventional Ileostomy.* Chicago, Year Book Medical Publishers, 1984. (In press.)
52. Bess M.A., Adson M.A., Elveback L.R., et al.: Rectal cancer following colectomy for polyposis. *Arch. Surg.* 115:460, 1980.
53. Adson M.A., Farnell M.B.: Ileorectostomy: clinical results and current role, in Dozois R.R., *Alternatives to Conventional Ileostomy.* Chicago, Year Book Medical Publishers, 1984. (In press.)
54. McGregor J.K., Bacon H.E.: The surgical management of carcinoma of the mid and upper rectum; abdominoperineal proctosigmoidectomy without abdominal colostomy and with sphincter muscle preservation: a critical anaylsis of 699 cases. *Arch. Surg.* 85:807, 1962.
55. Corman M.L., Heggelt R.C.: Carcinoma of the anal canal. *Surg. Gynecol. Obstet.* 145:674, 1977.
56. Stearns M.W., Quan S.H.Q.: Epidermoid carcinoma of the anorectum. *Surg. Gynecol. Obstet.* 131:953, 1970.
57. Beahrs O.H., Wilson S.H.: Carcinoma of the anus. *Ann. Surg.* 184:422, 1976.
58. Morson B.C.: Pathology and results of treatment of squamous cell carcinoma of the anal region in neoplastic disease at various sites, in Dukes C.E. (ed.): *Cancer of the Rectum.* Baltimore, Williams & Wilkins, 1960.
59. O'Brien P.H., Jeannette J.M., Wallace K.M., et al.: Epidermoid carcinoma of the anus. *Surg. Gynecol. Obstet.* 155:745, 1982.
60. Schneider T.C., Schulte W.J.: Management of carcinoma of the anal canal. *Surgery* 90:729, 1981.
61. Beart R.W., Jr.: Rare anal tumors. Unpublished review, 1980.
62. Morson B.C.: Pathology and results of treatment of cancer of the anal region. *Proc. Royal Soc. Med.* (Suppl.) 52:117.
63. Nigro N.D., Vaithevicius U.K., Considen B.: Combined therapy for cancer of the anal canal: a preliminary report. *Dis. Colon Rectum* 354–56, 1974.
64. Stearns M.W., Urmacker C., Steinberg S.S., et al.: Cancer of the anal canal. *Curr. Prob. Cancer,* 4:12, 1980.
65. Bowman B.M., O'Connell M.J., Moertel C.G., et al.: Cancer of the anal canal: the Mayo Clinic experience, 1950–1976. (Accepted for publication.) *Cancer,* 1984.
66. Mason J.K., Helwig E.B.: Anorectal melanoma. *Cancer* 39, 1966.
67. Chiu Y.S., Unni K.K., Beart R.W., Jr.: Malignant melanoma of the anorectum. *Dis. Colon Rectum* 23:122, 1980.
68. Baskies A.M., Sugarbaker E.V., Chretien P.B., et al.: Anorectal melanoma: the role of posterior pelvic exentoration. *Dis. Colon Rectum* 772, 1982.
69. Wolff B.G., Beart R.W., Jr.: Anal and perirectal problems; anal tumors, *Textbook of Gastroenterology.* Saunders WB, London, 1984. (In press.)
70. Devine R., Beart R.W., Jr., Wolff B.G.: Lymphomatous involvement of the rectum. Submitted for publication 1984.
71. Papillon J.: Intracavitary irradiation of early rectal cancer for cure: a series of 186 cases. *Cancer* 36:696, 1975.
72. Salvatti E.P., Rubin B.J.: Electrocoagulation as primary therapy for rectal carcinoma. *Am. J. Surg.* 132:583, 1976.

73. Beahrs O.H.: Low anterior resection for cancer of the rectosigmoid and rectum. *Surg. Clin. North Am.* 47:971, 1967.
74. Vandertoll D.J., Beahrs O.H.: Carcinoma of the rectum and low sigmoid: evaluation of anterior resection of 1,766 favorable lesions. *Arch. Surg.* 90:793, 1965.
75. Goligher J.C., Lee P.W.G., Simkins K.C., et al.: A controlled comparison of one and two layer techniques for suture of high and low colorectal anastomosis. *Br. J. Surg.* 64:609, 1977.
76. D'Allaine S., Localio S.A., Baron B.: Abdominotranssacral resection in anastomosis for midrectal cancer. *Ann. Surg.* 178:540, 1973.
77. Gunderson L.L., Sosin H.: Areas of failure found at reoperation (second or symptomatic look) following "curative surgery" for adenocarcinoma of the rectum: clinical pathologic correlation and implications for adjuvant therapy. *Cancer* 34:1278, 1974.
78. Localio S.A., Nealon W., Newall J., et al.: Adjuvant postoperative radiation therapy for Dukes C adenocarcinoma of the rectum. *Ann. Surg.* 198:18, 1983.
79. Stearns M.W., Jr., Schottenfled D.: Techniques for surgical management of colon cancer. *Cancer* 165:28, 1971.
80. Akwari O.E., Kelly K.A.: Anterior resection for adenocarcinoma of the distal large bowel. *Am. J. Surg.* 139:88, 1980.
81. Goligher J.C., Graham N.G., De Dombal F.T.: Anastomotic dehiscence after anterior resection of the rectum and sigmoid. *Br. J. Surg.* 57:109, 1970.
82. McLachlin A.D., Olsson L.S., Pitt D.F.: Anterior anastomosis of the rectosigmoid colon: an experimental study. *Surgery* 80:306, 1976.
83. Akwari O.E., Kelly K.A.: Anterior resection for adenocarcinoma of the distal large bowel. *Am. J. Surg.* 139:88, 1980.
84. Suzuki H., Matsumoto K., Amano S., et al.: Anorectal pressure and rectal compliance after low anterior resection. *Br. J. Surg.* 67:655, 1980.
85. Beart R.W., Jr., Kelly K.A.: Randomized prospective evaluation of the EEA stapler for colorectal anastomosis. *Am. J. Surg.* 141:143, 1981.
86. Brennen S.S., Pickford I.R., Evans M., et al.: Staples or sutures for colonic anastomosis: a controlled clinical trial. *Br. J. Surg.* 69:222, 1982.
87. Grafner H., Fredlund P., Olsson S., et al.: Protective colostomy and low anterior resection of the rectum using the EEA stapling instrument: a randomized study. *Dis. Colon Rectum* 26:87, 1983.
88. Rosen C.B., Beart R.W., Jr., Ilstrup D.M.: Local recurrence of rectal carcinoma after hand-sewn and stapled anastomoses. Presented at the American Society of Colon and Rectal Surgeons Convention, New Orleans, May 6–10, 1984.
89. Ballantyne G.H.: The experimental basis of intestinal suturing. *Dis. Colon Rectum* 27:61, 1984.
90. Black B.M., Walls J.T.: Combined abdominal endorectal resection: appraisal of a pull-thru procedure. *Surg. Clin. North Am.* 47:977, 1967.
91. Bacon H.E.: Present status of pull-thru sphincter preserving procedure. *Cancer* 28:296, 1971.
92. Postlethwait R.W.: An appraisal of operations for rectal carcinoma Monogr. Surg. Sci. 4:217, 1967.

93. Kennedy J.T., McComish D., Bennett R.C., et al.: Abdominoanal pull-thru resection of the rectum. *Br. J. Surg.* 57:589, 1970.
94. Parks A.G., Percey J.P.: Resection and sutured coloanal anastomosis for rectal carcinoma. *Br. J. Surg.* 69:301, 1982.
95. Lean R.H.S., Parks A.G.: Function of the anal sphincters following coloanal anastomosis. *Br. J. Surg.* 64:596, 1977.
96. Beart R.W., Jr.: Personal communication.

NMR: The New Frontier in Diagnostic Radiology

J. BRUCE KNEELAND, B. C. P. LEE, J. P.
WHALEN, R. J. R. KNOWLES, AND P. T. CAHILL

*The New York Hospital Cornell Medical Center, 525 East 68th Street,
New York, New York*

THE PHYSICS of nuclear magnetic resonance (NMR) imaging has a surprisingly long history. In 1924, W. Pauli postulated the existence of nuclear magnetism to explain the presence of hyperfine structures in atomic spectra.[1] During the 1930s, I. I. Rabi and collaborators performed magnetic resonance experiments on molecular beams.[2] In the 1940s, groups headed by E. M. Purcell and F. Bloch independently obtained NMR signals from liquids and solids.[3, 4] By the 1960s, NMR had become a powerful method for analyzing molecular structure in organic chemistry. In 1973, P. C. Lauterbur produced the first NMR images.[5] Work on nuclear magnetism has already yielded two Nobel Prizes and may soon yield more.

Theory of NMR Imaging

NMR uses a strong magnetic field and radiofrequency (rf) waves to obtain two-dimensional images of the body in any plane.[6–8] Basically, four components are necessary for the production of such images: (1) magnetic nuclei, (2) a strong static magnetic field, (3) coils to transmit and receive rf waves, and (4) magnetic gradients (small magnetic fields with known, carefully controlled spatial variations). The actual image is re-

37

0065-3411/84/0018-0037-0066-$04.00

constructed from the observed rf signals by use of a computer in a manner similar to that already made familiar by computerized tomography (CT).

NUCLEAR MAGNETISM

Only nuclei with an odd number of neutrons or protons possess a net spin with significant nuclear magnetism. Magnetic nuclei of particular importance in biologic systems include hydrogen (H), carbon(^{13}C), fluorine (^{19}F), sodium (^{23}Na), and phosphorus (^{31}P). Because of the high mobile proton (hydrogen) content of biologic tissues, most NMR imaging to date has been proton imaging.

THE STATIC MAGNETIC FIELD

When magnetic nuclei are placed in a strong magnetic field, they tend to align themselves along the direction of this field. Because the magnetic nuclei have intrinsic spin (with associated dipole moments), they may be conceptualized as precessing about the magnetic field lines like tiny spinning tops or gyroscopes (Fig 1). The rate at which this precession occurs is described by the Larmor equation:

$$w = gB$$

where w is frequency, g is a constant (the magnetogyric ratio, which is different for each different type of nucleus), and B is the static magnetic field strength. For example, in a field of 1.0 T (1 tesla = 10,000 gauss, symbolized as B), protons precess at a Larmor frequency of 42.57 MHz (1 megahertz = 1,000,000 cycles per second), while phosphorus nuclei precess at 17.24 MHz. (Note that the earth's magnetic field is approximately 0.5 B.)

RADIOFREQUENCY ENERGY EXCHANGE

Magnetic nuclei in a known static magnetic field absorb and emit energy at their Larmor frequency. Short pulses of rf energy push the spinning nuclei away from the direction of the magnetic field lines. For example, a 90-degree pulse causes the nuclei to rotate their axes perpendicular to the static magnetic

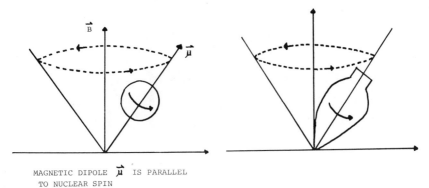

MAGNETIC DIPOLE $\vec{\mu}$ IS PARALLEL
TO NUCLEAR SPIN

Fig 1.—*Left,* association between nuclear spin and nuclear magnetic moment is illustrated. *Right,* analogy between magnetic moments in a magnetic field and a spinning top in a gravitational field is presented to explain precession.

field (Fig 2,A). A 180-degree pulse causes the nuclei to rotate until they are antiparallel to the magnetic field direction (Fig 2,B). It is the component of the nuclear magnetization perpendicular to the static magnetic field that provides the rf signal from which images can be constructed.

After magnetic nuclei have been tipped away from the direction of the static magnetic field, they tend to reorient themselves gradually in the direction of the field and to spread out in the transverse plane. The rate of disappearance of the perpendicular component of the nuclear magnetism (and hence of the rf signal) depends on two relaxation times: T_1 and T_2. T_1 measures the rate at which the nuclei realign along the direction of the static magnetic field (Fig 3,A). T_2 measures the rate at which the nuclei lose synchronization with each other and fan out perpendicular to the static magnetic field (Fig 3,B). Both T_1 and T_2 tell us something about the relationship between the nuclear spins and their local environment. Thus the rf signal contains implicit biochemical and physiologic information. In an NMR imaging system, the observed strength of the rf signal emitted from any volume of matter (typically, $1 \times 1 \times 8$ mm) is a complex function of the number of magnetic nuclei in that volume (nuclear density), any flow of nuclei in or out of the measured volume, and the average relaxation times in that volume. The exact functional form of the rf signal in turn depends on the type and timing of the rf pulses. Two com-

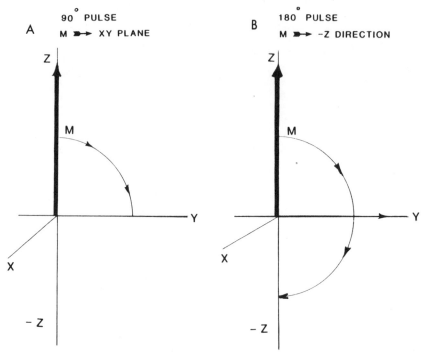

Fig 2.—A, effects of a 90-degree radiofrequency pulse on the net magnetic moment, presented diagrammatically. B, effects of a 180-degree radiofrequency pulse.

monly used pulse sequences are the spin-echo sequence (a 90-degree pulse followed by a 180-degree pulse) and the inversion-recovery sequence (a 180-degree pulse followed by a 90-degree pulse). The high soft tissue contrasts characteristic of NMR images are produced by differences in rf signal strength.

MAGNETIC GRADIENTS

Since for a given nuclear species (e.g., protons) the Larmor equation predicts a unique relationship between frequency and magnetic field strength, the effect of introducing magnetic field gradients (i.e., small systematic changes on the order of 0.5 B/cm) is to make each spatial location correspond to a different Larmor frequency (Fig 4). Thus by measuring the rf signal intensity at different frequencies or phases, one can distinguish

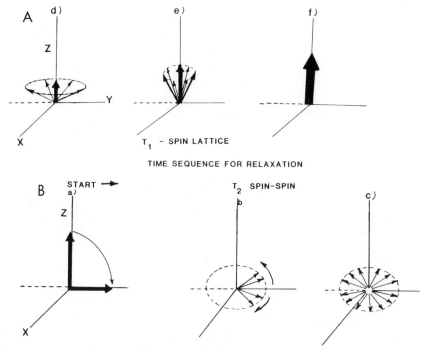

Fig 3.—A, magnetic moments that have already relaxed by T_2 (T_2 is always $\leq T_1$) relax longitudinally by T_1 mechanisms. **B,** magnetic moments relax transversely by T_2 mechanisms alone.

these signals and assign them to different three-dimensional spatial locations in the volume being imaged.

CHEMICAL SHIFT IMAGING AND SPECTROSCOPY

It is worth noting at this point that not all local variations in magnetic field strength are applied by external magnetic gradients. Some very important changes in magnetic field strength result from the chemical environment of the nuclear spins. For example, in a simple compound such as ethyl alcohol (CH_3-CH_2-OH), the proton associated with the oxygen experiences a slightly different magnetic field strength than those near the carbon, and there is even a difference between protons attached to the carbon with three hydrogens and those attached to the carbon with only two hydrogens (Fig 5). Such slight frequency shifts produced by neighboring atoms are the basis for the structural determinations made by organic chemists, as noted above. The in vivo imaging of these so-called chemical shifts in frequency and the performing of detailed spectroscopic analyses in arbitrarily selected volumes for various magnetic nuclei are exciting possibilities that are currently active areas of research.

IMAGE GATING

One can eliminate physiologic motions (i.e., cardiac, respiratory, or both) by physiologic gating. In such a technique, one acquires NMR data only at a fixed time interval relative to the cardiac or respiratory cycle. This can greatly improve image quality by removing motion artifacts, but the acquisition time is increased.

Fig 4.—*Left,* the magnetic field is constant, and two identical vials have identical Larmor frequencies. *Right,* there is a linear magnetic gradient (increasing from left to right), and two identical vials have Larmor frequencies that depend on their positions in the field (frequency A is less than frequency B).

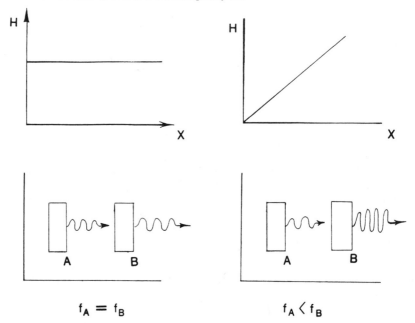

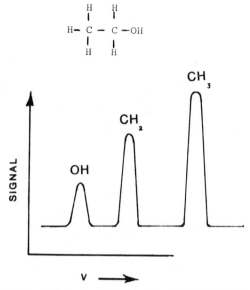

Fig 5.—Proton spectrum for ethanol (CH₃-CH₂-OH).

Measuring Flow

Because macroscopic flow of nuclei changes the rf signal strength measured from any volume, flow acts as a sort of natural contrast agent, and thus many details of vascular anatomy can be studied without invasive techniques. True noninvasive quantitation of blood, urine, and even cerebrospinal fluid (CSF) flow is a very exciting possibility. Several different schemes for measuring nonturbulent and turbulent flow have been attempted in vitro and in vivo for vessels greater than 2 mm in diameter,[9, 10] but further research is still needed to validate in vivo flow studies.

Magnetic Contrast Agents

Electrons possess magnetic moments more than a thousand times stronger than nuclear magnetic moments, and it is through these moments that ions or molecules with any unpaired electrons can greatly alter nuclear relaxation times and thus change the NMR signal. Currently, two different sources of unpaired electrons are being explored in attempts to develop magnetic contrast agents.[11, 12] First, there are paramagnetic ions such as manganese, gadolinium, chromium, and iron, which are, in general, rather toxic and must be chelated to reduce toxicity. [Thus far, iron (Fig 6) is unique in that ferric ammonium citrate solutions have been used directly to improve gastrointestinal contrast.] Such ions can be chelated to compounds such as EDTA and DPTA or to considerably more specific agents such as monoclonal antibodies. Second, free radicals such as the nitroxide stable free radical also provide unpaired electrons to change tissue contrast. Unfortunately, free radicals are potentially carcinogenic so that much testing will be necessary before agents incorporating them can be made available for human use. Signal intensities from tissues have been increased by as much as a factor of 10 through the use of magnetic contrast agents.[13]

POTENTIAL HAZARDS OF NMR

Considerable epidemiologic and experimental work has failed to reveal any hazards associated with the static magnetic field strengths, changing magnetic fields (gradients), or rf energy levels currently used in NMR imaging.[14, 15] At present, the only potential hazards involve magnetic objects brought into the vicinity of the magnet or used as surgical implants. Strong magnetic fields may turn ferromagnetic objects into dangerous projectiles. It is therefore essential that proper security measures to exclude such objects from the vicinity of the

Fig 6.—A, patient was imaged without contrast material. B, patient was imaged following the administration of a dilute solution of ferric ammonium citrate (Geritol). In the non-contrast study (A), the liver and stomach *(st)* are virtually indistinguishable, but in B these organs are readily separated.

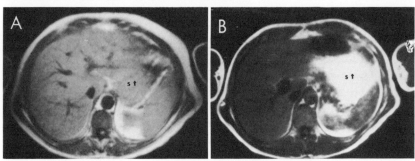

magnet be enforced. Changing magnetic fields may induce currents in the leads of cardiac pacemakers and thus precipitate cardiac arrhythmias. In addition, the static magnetic field may switch cardiac pacemakers from the demand to the fixed mode. Hence, patients with cardiac pacemakers should not be scanned.[16] Moreover, the FDA recommends that magnetic fields as low as 5 B be posted with warning signs for pacemaker users. Finally, magnetic fields may exert excessive torque on vascular clips that happen to be magnetic.[17] At present, no one with aneurysm clips should be scanned unless it has been established that the clips are nonmagnetic.

Clinical NMR Imaging of the CNS

CT scanning is well established as a useful tool in the diagnosis of neurologic diseases. There are, however, some important limitations inherent in CT technology. First, CT imaging is based on the differential absorption of x-rays, and for the common range of CT x-ray energies, observed differences in x-ray absorption result almost exclusively from local variations in electron density. Thus, CT image contrast is essentially produced by variations in a single parameter. Second, the geometry of the CT scanning process restricts imaging basically to tranverse sections (although some coronal sections can be obtained with great difficulty). Because of this limitation, images in other planes must be calculated from transverse sections and normally have reduced spatial resolution with increased noise. Third, the juxtaposition of skull and CNS soft tissues often produces image degradation through streak artifacts, especially in the posterior fossa and sella regions. NMR imaging, on the other hand, offers distinct advantages in all three aspects. First, NMR image contrast results from many parameters: mobile hydrogen density, flow, and T_1 and T_2 relaxation times. This affords a greater potential for soft tissue discrimination. Second, the NMR scanning process can directly yield high resolution images in coronal and sagittal planes as well as in the transverse plane. Third, since cortical bone is transparent to NMR, there are no associated image streak artifacts.

To realize the full advantages of greater soft tissue discrimination and multiplanar imaging, multiple pulse sequences must be used. The same lesion, however, may be visualized very differently with different pulse sequences (i.e., abnormalities may be darker than normal tissue for some pulse sequences, lighter for others, and isodense for still others). Determination of optimal pulse sequences is currently an area of active research.[18–22]

The published literature and our own experience indicate that NMR is the method of choice for the diagnosis of multiple sclerosis.[22] Indications for NMR scanning of other CNS abnormalities are not yet as clearly established.[23–32] On the basis of our experience with a 0.5 T Technicare superconducting system, we have grouped suspected lesions into three categories: those in which NMR is superior to CT, those in which NMR may potentially be more informative than CT, and those in which CT is currently superior to NMR (Table 1).

WHEN NMR IS THE METHOD OF CHOICE

BRAIN STEM TUMORS.—NMR accurately delineates intrinsic expansion of the brain stem from tumor involvement, both in cases where CT is uninformative because of artifacts and in cases where CT does suggest the diagnosis (Fig 7).[33] NMR spatial resolution is similar to that obtained from CT scans using injected intrathecal contrast material.

TABLE 1.—NMR VERSUS CT

CONDITION	NMR SUPERIOR TO CT	NMR PROBABLY SUPERIOR TO CT	CT SUPERIOR TO NMR	NO. OF STUDIES
Multiple scelerosis	35	3	. . .	38
Brain stem tumor	15 (10)*	. . .	. . .	15
Other PF tumors	5	3	1	9
Other PF lesions	6	9	2 (2)†	17
Craniocervical junct.	6	. . .	. . .	6
Cerebral trauma	2 (2)*	3	. . .	5
Spinal canal	6	. . .	2	8
Hemisphere tumors	7 (7)*	22	2 (2)†	31
Other supratent. tumors	. . .	4	. . .	4
Other supratent. lesions	6	7	6 (1)†	19
Juxta/suprasellar tumors	3	32	8‡	43
Lumbar disk disease	—	2	8	10
Totals	91	85	29	205

*Lesions missed on CT.
†Lesions missed on NMR.
‡Microadenomas.

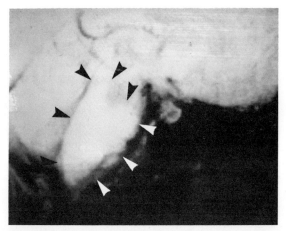

Fig 7.—Sagittal spin-echo image of brain stem glioma. Enlarged pons and medulla (arrowheads) have increased signal intensity.

OTHER POSTERIOR FOSSA TUMORS.—Cerebellar hemispheres and convexity meningiomas are clearly identified on NMR scans. The patency of the venous sinuses can sometimes be evaluated (Fig 8). Cerebellopontine angle tumors are better visualized than with CT. In addition, the degree of brain stem compression can be accurately evaluated.[33, 34] It is also possible

Fig 8 (left).—Axial spin-echo image of meningioma. Tumor (arrows) and surrounding edema (arrowheads) both have high signal intensity.

Fig 9 (right).—Sagittal partial saturation image of arachnoid cyst. Cyst extends from posterior fossa into upper cervical spine, causing compression of cerebellum (arrowheads).

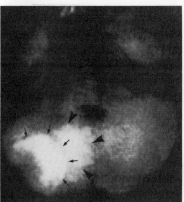
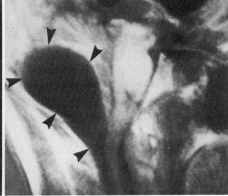

to differentiate hematoma from calcification, since the latter produces no NMR signal.

OTHER POSTERIOR FOSSA LESIONS.—The site of aqueductal stenosis is well delineated by NMR. NMR also allows arachnoid cysts to be differentiated from cysts with other etiologies (Fig 9). Furthermore, nonsurgical lesions such as degeneration of the cerebellum and brain stem are well visualized on NMR scans.[35]

CRANIOCERVICAL JUNCTION LESIONS.—Chiari I malformations are optimally seen in sagittal sections (Fig 10).[36] Basilar impression, atlantoaxial dislocation secondary to trauma, and rheumatoid arthritis are also ideally evaluated through sagittal images.

CEREBRAL TRAUMA.—NMR is more accurate than CT in visualizing extracerebral and intracerebral hematomas and contusions (Fig 11).[37] NMR is particularly useful in evaluating the postconcussion syndrome when CT scans are normal. Unfortunately, it is not yet possible to scan many acutely traumatized patients, owing to the presence of various life support devices (respirators, traction frames, etc.).

SPINAL CORD LESIONS.—CT scans of spinal cord lesions are

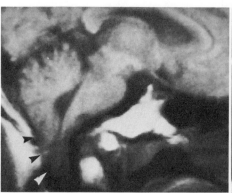
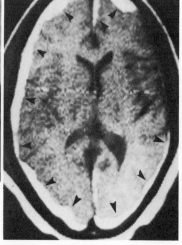

Fig 10 (above).—Sagittal partial saturation image of Chiari I malformation. Cerebellar tonsils extend to upper cervical level and are inseparable from the spinal cord *(arrowheads)*.

Fig 11 (right).—Axial spin-echo image of head trauma. Subdural hematoma is seen as high signal intensity *(arrowheads)*. CT scan was normal.

generally nondiagnostic unless the lesions cause enlargement of the canal and extend outside the exit foramina. The spatial resolution of NMR is comparable to that of myelography, so that lesions are separable into epidural, intradural, extramedullary, and intramedullary locations (Fig 12). In addition, syrinx cavities are sometimes visualized.[38, 39]

WHEN NMR IS PROBABLY SUPERIOR TO CT

SUPRATENTORIAL TUMORS.—CT scans generally provide accurate diagnosis of primary and metastatic tumors of the cerebral hemispheres since these regions are usually free of bone artifacts; however, tumors which do not cause distortion of the ventricles and are isodense with normal brain are not seen on CT. A significant number of such tumors have been observed on NMR in our study (Fig 13). Although it is often not possible to differentiate the tumor from surrounding edema with NMR, we believe that NMR will be the method of choice for evaluating clinically suspected tumors.[40]

Meningiomas are clearly visualized with NMR and are usually distinguishable from adjacent edema. Both extrinsic and intrinsic tumors can be more fully evaluated by NMR, in which

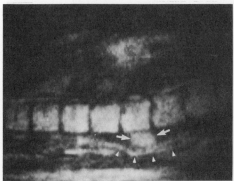
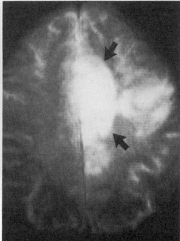

Fig 12 (above).—Sagittal spin-echo image of meningioma. There is an intradural extramedullary tumor *(arrows)* posterior to the conus medullaris *(arrowheads)*.

Fig 13 (right).—Axial spin-echo image of glioma. Note area of high signal intensity *(arrows)*. CT scan was normal.

the relationship of the tumor to important regions of normal function such as the motor and speech centers can be delineated (Fig 14).

OTHER SUPRATENTORIAL LESIONS.—Arteriovenous malformations, giant aneurysms, abcesses, arachnoid cysts, herpes simplex encephalitis, disseminated lupus erythematosus, and infarcts are normally well visualized on CT. Such lesions are equally well evaluated by NMR without requiring intravenous contrast materials.[41-45]

Fig 14 (top).—Lateral partial saturation image of glioma. Note mass in parietal lobe above sylvian fissure, with displacement of branches of the middle cerebral arteries *(arrowheads)*.

Fig 15 (bottom).—Sagittal inversion-recovery image of sella tumor. Suprasellar extension of tumor causes compression of optic chiasm and nerves *(arrowheads)*.

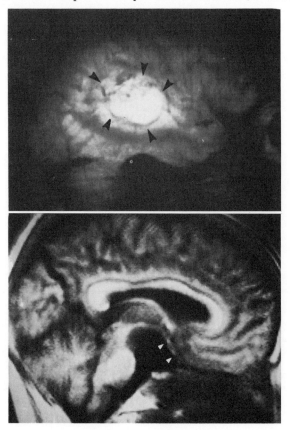

SELLAR/JUXTASELLAR LESIONS.—Thin section CT scanning with multiple plane reformatting currently provides accurate evaluation of suprasellar and parasellar extension of intrasellar tumors; however, the relationship of these tumors to the optic chiasm and third ventricle can be seen on NMR (Fig 15). In addition, NMR also demonstrates whether the carotid arteries are patent (Fig 16).

Craniopharyngiomas, on the other hand, are often not well visualized on CT scans since they have decreased attenuation and are not enhanced with injected contrast. NMR demonstrates these lesions clearly because the cholesterol content gives rise to extremely intense signals for both the spin-echo and inversion-recovery sequences (Fig 17).

OTHER SUPRASELLAR TUMORS.—Optic chiasm gliomas are visualized by NMR, and the extent of tumor involvement is better determined by NMR than by CT. Hypothalamic tumors are seen equally well on NMR and on CT.

WHEN NMR IS NOT AS USEFUL AS CT

LUMBAR DISK LESIONS.—NMR is currently less accurate than CT in the diagnosis of herniated lumbar disks because the spatial resolution of NMR in the body is currently not as good as

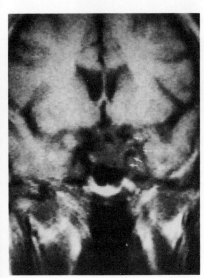

Fig 16.—Coronal partial saturation image of meningioma. Right carotid is normal, but left carotid (though still present) is narrowed by tumor encasement (arrows).

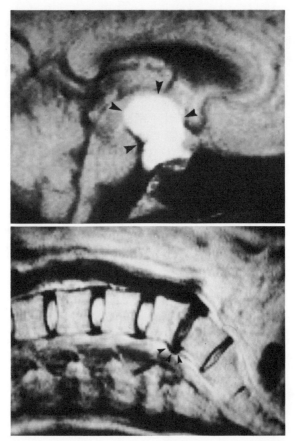

Fig 17 (top).—Sagittal partial saturation image of craniopharyngioma. Note suprasellar lesion of high signal intensity *(arrowheads)*. CT scan was normal.
Fig 18 (bottom).—Sagittal spin-echo image of disk herniation. Note low signal from L4-5 disk and compression of the subarachnoid space *(arrowheads)*.

CT (Fig 18).[32, 38, 39] (This situation, though, may change drastically with the introduction of surface coils.) NMR, however, is useful in postoperative cases where disk recurrence is difficult to evaluate by CT. NMR is also useful in diagnosing whether an intervertebral disk is abnormal: normal disks produce an intense NMR signal, while degenerated and herniated disks both produce markedly decreased signal intensity. Furthermore, NMR may prove useful in evaluating the extent of involvement for disk infections.

MISSED LESIONS.—Very small lesions may be missed on NMR. In our series, one very small vascular malformation of the brain stem and two small supratentorial calcified lesions were not visualized on NMR. In addition, two presumed cerebral infarcts were not seen (probably because of the long interval between initial diagnosis and NMR examination).

Clinical NMR Imaging in the Body

Considerable experience in body imaging at different magnetic field strengths has already been acquired at several centers throughout the world, including our own.[46-77] These studies have yielded much preliminary information on normal conditions and on numerous pathologic entities; however, in most cases the results are insufficient to permit firm conclusions to be made regarding the efficacy of NMR relative to other imaging modalities.

In general, the spatial resolution of NMR images in the body is less than for NMR images of the head and less than for current CT images of the body. (This situation, though, may change drastically with the introduction of surface coils which receive NMR signals from only limited regions of the body but which offer much higher spatial resolution. To date, three manufacturers have produced high resolution images from prototype surface coils.) In addition, the long data acquisition times currently required for body imaging (5–30 minutes) result in loss of detail from motion artifacts caused by physiologic movements (i.e., cardiac, respiratory, and peristaltic), even though this problem can be ameliorated by using gated data acquisition. NMR imaging, however, does offer the advantages of superior soft tissue discrimination, better delineation of vascular structures (because bulk flow directly alters the NMR signal), equal resolution in three mutually perpendicular planes (transverse, sagittal, and coronal), and the absence of streak artifacts such as those associated with beam hardening in CT.

THORAX (EXCLUDING HEART)

The absence or reduction of NMR signal from vessels in the chest gives NMR a significant advantage over CT in the evaluation of hilar and mediastinal masses and lymphadenopathy

(Fig 19).[46-49] NMR may also be more sensitive than CT in detecting invasion of the chest wall by parenchymal masses,[48] even though inferior spatial resolution and the lack of signal from calcifications render NMR less sensitive than CT in the detection of pulmonary nodules.[46] The reliability of NMR for distinguishing benign and malignant pulmonary nodules on the basis of quantitative T_1 and T_2 relaxation time measurements has yet to be fully explored.[49] At our institution, we are currently evaluating the ability of NMR to discriminate between edema, inflammatory infiltrate, and pulmonary infarction in a canine model.

The female breast has been imaged in a limited number of

Fig 19 (top).—Transverse section through superior mediastinum. Note black appearance of great vessels. The medium-intensity round structure posteromedial to the right innominate vein *(arrow)* is an enlarged lymph node involved by metastatic tumor.

Fig 20 (bottom).—Transverse section through heart. Note that chambers and vessels are black. In addition, the proximal coronary arteries are visualized *(rca,* right coronary artery; *lad,* left anterior descending coronary artery).

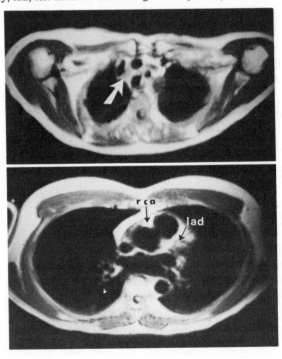

patients.[50, 51] Although it did not prove possible to distinguish between benign and malignant disease on the basis of T_1 relaxation times,[50] it was felt that it was possible to discriminate between most benign and malignant lesions on the basis of configuration using criteria similar to those used in mammography.[51]

CARDIOVASCULAR SYSTEM

Gated NMR studies of the heart acquire NMR signals only during a fixed time interval relative to the cardiac cycle but sum data from many cardiac cycles. Such studies have produced excellent displays of cardiac anatomy, including valves, papillary muscles, proximal coronary arteries, and pericardium (Fig 20).[52-54]

NMR imaging of canine hearts with experimentally induced infarcts has revealed significant increases in T_2 relaxation times for the infarcted myocardium.[54] In man, the post-myocardial infarction complications of intraventricular thrombus formation and ventricular aneurysm have been demonstrated.[55] In addition, NMR imaging has demonstrated great potential for the evaluation of congenital heart disease.[55]

The natural contrast supplied by flowing blood permits good visualization of vascular abnormalities such as aneurysms, aortic dissections, thrombosis, and atherosclerotic plaques (Fig 21).[54, 56] In a small number of cases, NMR imaging has demonstrated the patency of coronary artery bypass grafts.[56]

In spite of the impressive results to date, however, NMR may have its greatest impact on the diagnosis and management of cardiovascular diseases through its potential ability to measure flow and to evaluate ischemic tissue by ^{31}P spectroscopy.[57]

GASTROINTESTINAL SYSTEM

The GI system has proved to be one of the most difficult regions to image because of image degradation from respiratory and (to a lesser degree) peristaltic motion.

A variety of benign and malignant, primary and metastatic liver tumors have been imaged by NMR.[58-60] The evaluation of liver tumors by NMR appears to be comparable to CT evaluations at this time, although NMR gives better definition of the

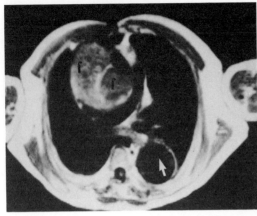
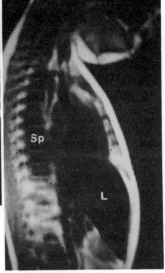

Fig 21 (above).—Transverse section through the heart. Dissection present in ascending (*f,* false lumen with thrombus) and descending aorta is readily seen. Note intimal flap in descending aorta *(arrow).*

Fig 22 (right).—Sagittal section through midline chest and abdomen. Note dark appearance of liver *(L)* and vertebral bodies *(Sp)* due to iron deposition.

relationship of the mass to the vasculature of the liver.[60] NMR has also been used to image a number of nonneoplastic liver diseases in both animals[61] and man.[58, 62] Hepatitis has been noted to produce increased NMR signal intensity and prolonged T_1 and T_2 relaxation times.[60–62] Rather surprisingly, neither cirrhosis nor fatty infiltration has demonstrated any measurable effect on signal intensity or relaxation times.[62] Hemochromatosis, on the other hand, causes a marked reduction in NMR signal intensity that correlates well with iron concentration, as has been demonstrated in animal experiments (Fig 22).[61]

NMR can assess the ability of the gallbladder to concentrate bile (an ability impaired in the presence of chronic cholecystitis) and the ability of the gallbladder to empty following cholecystogogue administration.[63] Irrespective of composition, the majority of gallstones (83%) produce no NMR signal,[64] but gallstones may still be visualized as regions of low intensity ("filling defects") in the high signal returned by bile.[63]

The pancreas is also a difficult organ to image with NMR.

One recent study reported visualization of the normal pancreas in only about 60% of the patients (Fig 23).[65] These results, however, may improve with the use of respiratory gating. Pancreatic neoplasms greater than 3 cm in diameter have been imaged,[65] together with dilation of the common duct. (Smaller islet cell tumors may potentially be visualized because of the increased signal intensity of these tumors.) Enlargement of the pancreas and infiltration of the surrounding soft tissue planes have been demonstrated in patients with acute pancreatitis, and in one case pancreatitis was detected in a patient with a

Fig 23 (top).—Transverse section through normal pancreas *(p)*.

Fig 24 (bottom).—Transverse section through normal adrenal glands. Note darker appearance of renal medulla, especially on left *(ladr, left adrenal)*.

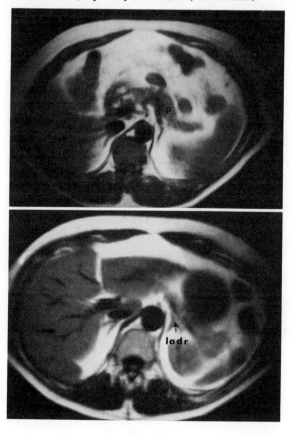

normal CT scan on the basis of altered T_1 and T_2 relaxation times.[65] In addition, pseudocysts larger than 1.5 cm have been visualized.[65]

Portal hypertension has been found to increase the NMR signal intensity and to prolong both T_1 and T_2 relaxation times in the spleen.[66] Collateral vessels are also readily demonstrated.[66] In addition, the potential of NMR to measure blood flow in the portal system may have a significant effect on the management of those patients in whom shunt surgery is contemplated or has already been performed.

GENITOURINARY SYSTEM

Although not properly a part of the GU system, the adrenal glands are usually grouped with the kidneys because of their physical proximity (Fig 24). Benign and malignant, primary and metastatic adrenal tumors as well as adrenal hyperplasia have been imaged with NMR. The observed detection rate is comparable to that achieved with CT.[67] In addition, NMR offers the unique ability to differentiate cortex and medulla in at least some patients.[67] Whether or not this will prove clinically useful remains to be seen.

In the urinary tract, dilation of the collecting system is readily visualized on NMR. When dilation results from obstruction, normal corticomedullary differentiation is not seen.[68]

NMR appears comparable to CT in the detection of renal masses and in its ability to distinguish cystic from solid masses.[69] NMR is superior to CT in its ability to distinguish simple cysts from those complicated by hemorrhage.[69] Because of its multiplanar imaging capabilities, NMR is superior to CT in the evaluation of the extension of tumor, both intravascular and into adjacent structures. NMR has been demonstrated to be as effective as CT in the detection and evaluation of the extent of retroperitoneal fibrosis and superior to CT in the assessment of vascular involvement.[70]

In patients with renal transplants (Fig 25), NMR has been able to differentiate between acute rejection and ATN on the basis of differences in the corticomedullary differentiation.[71]

The only weakness of NMR in the assessment of renal disease is in its inability to directly detect calcifications, including calculi, except as the absence of signal.

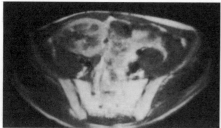
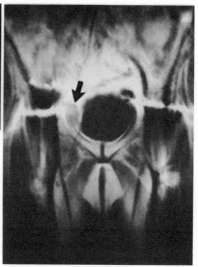

Fig 25 (above).—Transverse section through normally functioning renal transplant in the pelvis demonstrating excellent corticomedullary differentiation.
Fig 26 (right).—Coronal section through the pelvis illustrates a soft tissue mass to right of bladder *(arrow).* Abnormal appearance of image in the region of the femoral heads is due to presence of bilateral hip prostheses which rendered CT scan totally nondiagnostic.

NMR imaging in the pelvis is excellent, being greatly aided by the absence of respiratory motion. In the male pelvis, limited experience indicates that NMR is superior to CT in the detection and staging of prostatic and bladder neoplasms (Fig 26). This results primarily from superior soft tissue discrimination and multiplanar capabilities.[72] In the female pelvis, NMR appears to be a promising method for evaluating masses; however, the data are insufficient at this time to permit even a preliminary assessment of the role of NMR relative to the other imaging modalities.[73, 74]

MUSCULOSKELETAL SYSTEM

Patients with a variety of benign and malignant, primary and metastatic, osseous and soft tissue tumors have been imaged.[75, 76] NMR has demonstrated great sensitivity to the presence of intramedullary tumor (Fig 27).[75, 76] In a limited number of cases, NMR has shown greater sensitivity to the presence of acute osteomyelitis than has plain film radiography or radionuclide bone scans.[77] In addition, NMR has demonstrated definite abnormalities for avascular necrosis in cases with negative or equivocal plain films and bone scans.[76] The demonstration of injury to joints, such as meniscal tears, is difficult with the spa-

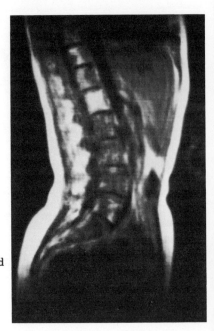

Fig 27.—Sagittal section through lumbosacral spine demonstrates mottled decrease in signal from marrow due to diffuse involvement by metastasis.

tial resolution of current NMR systems; however, the high spatial resolution demonstrated by recent surface coil images of the knee suggests the possible replacement of arthrography as the primary method of imaging joints.

Conclusions

Although still quite new, NMR imaging has already emerged as a safe, noninvasive, painless, and effective diagnostic modality requiring no ionizing radiation. Also, NMR appears already to have established itself as the method of choice for the examination of the brain and spinal cord (excluding herniated disks). Another area in which NMR excels is in the examination of the pelvis. The use of surface coils offers the promise of visualizing structures with resolution unobtainable by any other means.

In addition, NMR, with its superb visualization of vascular structures and potential ability to measure flow, may soon revolutionize the diagnosis of cardiovascular disease. Finally, NMR, through biochemically and physiologically based T_1 and

T_2 indices or through spectroscopy, may provide a means of monitoring therapeutic response so as to permit tailoring of treatment to the individual patient. In short, NMR is today probably at the same stage as the x-ray was in Roentgen's day.

Acknowledgments

The authors would like to thank especially the following Technicare staff for providing the strong support and extensive technical assistance so important in the joint venture between Technicare and New York Hospital of establishing the first successful 0.5 T NMR imaging system in a clinical setting: John Keller, David Kramer, Joseph Malysa, Joseph Mazella, Robert McCarthy, Thomas O'Brien, J. B. Richey, and Hong Yeung. In addition, we thank our technicians, Thomas Callahan and Richard Fischer, for their long hours, special care, and enthusiasm in running the system.

REFERENCES

1. Pauli W.: *Naturwissenschaften* 12:741, 1924.
2. Rabi I.I., Millman S., Kusch P., et al.: *Physical Rev.* 55:526, 1939.
3. Purcell E.M., Torrey H.C., Pound R.V.: Resonance absorption by nuclear magnetic moments in a solid. *Physical Rev.* 69:37, 1946.
4 Bloch F., Hansen W.W., Packard M.E.: Nuclear induction. *Physical Rev.* 69:127, 1946.
5. Lauterbur P.C.: Image formation by induced local interactions: Examples employing nuclear magnetic resonance. *Nature* 242:190, 1973.
6. Pykett I.L.: NMR imaging in Medicine. *Sci. Am.* 246(5):78–88, 1982.
7. Partain C.L., James A.E., Rollo F.D., et al. (eds.): *Nuclear Magnetic Resonance (NMR) Imaging*. Philadelphia, W.B. Saunders Co., 1983.
8. Mansfield P., Morris P.G.: *NMR Imaging in Biomedicine*. New York, Academic Press, 1982.
9. Moran P.R.: A flow velocity zeugmatographic interlace for NMR imaging in humans. *Magnetic Resonance Imaging* 1:197–203, 1982.
10. Singer J.R., Crooks L.E.: Nuclear magnetic resonance blood flow measurements in the human brain. *Science* 221:654–656, 1983.
11. Runge V.M., Clanton J.A., Lukehart C.M., et al.: Paramagnetic agents for contrast-enhanced NMR imaging: A review. *AJR* 141:1209–1215, 1983.
12. Brasch R.C.: Methods of contrast enhancement for NMR imaging and potential applications. *Radiology* 147:781–788, 1983.
13. Brady T.J.: Personal communication.
14. Budinger T.F.: Nuclear magnetic resonance (NMR) in vivo studies: Known thresholds for health effects. *J. Comput. Assist. Tomogr.* 5:800–811, 1981.

15. Saunders R.D., Orr J.S.: Biological effects of NMR in Partain C.L., et al. (eds.): *Nuclear Magnetic Resonance (NMR) Imaging*. Philadelphia, W.B. Saunders Co., 1983.
16. Pavlicek W., Geisinger M., Castle L., et al.: The effects of nuclear magnetic resonance on patients with cardiac pacemakers. *Radiology* 147:149–153, 1983.
17. New P.F.J., Rosen B.R., Brady T.J., et al.: Potential hazards and artifacts of ferromagnetic and nonferromagnetic surgical and dental materials and devices in nuclear magnetic resonance imaging. *Radiology* 147:139–148, 1983.
18. Crooks L.E., Mills C.M., Davis P.L., et al.: Visualization of cerebral and vascular abnormalities by NMR imaging: The effects of imaging parameters on contrast. *Radiology* 144:842–853, 1982.
19. Crooks L.E., Ortendahl D.A., Kaufman L., et al.: Clinical efficiency of nuclear magnetic resonance imaging. *Radiology* 146:123–128, 1983.
20. Hu K.W., Heindel W., Deimling S.E.: Nuclear magnetic resonance (NMR) tomography of the central nervous system: Comparison of two imaging sequences. *J. Comput. Assist. Tomogr.* 7:468–475, 1983.
21. Wehrli F.W., MacFall, Newton T.H.: Parameters determining the appearance of NMR images, in Newton T.H., Potts D.G. (eds.): *Modern Neuroradiology*. Vol. 2: *Advanced Imaging Techniques*. San Anselmo, Clavadel Press, 1983.
22. Young I.R., Randell C.P., Kaplan P.W., et al.: Nuclear magnetic resonance (NMR) imaging in white matter disease of the brain using spin-echo sequences. *J. Comput. Assist. Tomogr.* 7:290–294, 1983.
23. Hawkes R.C., Holland G.N., Moore W.S., et al.: Nuclear magnetic (NMR) tomography of the brain: A preliminary clinical assessment with demonstration of pathology. *J. Comput. Assist. Tomogr.* 4:577–586, 1980.
24. Doyle F.H., Gore J.C., Pennock J.M., et al.: Imaging of the brain by nuclear magnetic resonance. *Lancet* 1:53–57, 1981.
25. Bydder G.M., Steiner R.E.: NMR imaging of the brain. *Neuroradiology* 23:231–240, 1982.
26. Young I.R., Bailes D.R., Burl M., et al.: Initial clinical evaluation of the whole body nuclear magnetic resonance (NMR) tomography. *J. Comput. Assist. Tomogr.* 6:1–18, 1982.
27. Bydder G.M., Steiner R.E., Young I.R., et al.: Clinical NMR imaging of the brain: 140 cases. *AJR* 139:215–236, 1982.
28. Crooks L., Arakawa M., Hoenninger J., et al.: Nuclear magnetic resonance whole body imager operating at 3.5 KGauss. *Radiology* 143:169–174, 1982.
29. Steiner R.E.: The Hammersmith clinical experience with nuclear magnetic resonance. *Clin. Radiol.* 34:13–23, 1983.
30. Worthington B.S.: Clinical prospects of nuclear magnetic resonance. *Clin. Radiol.* 34:3–12, 1983.
31. Brant-Zawadzki M., Davis P.L., Crooks L.E., et al.: NMR demonstration of cerebral abnormalities: Comparison with CT. *AJNR* 4:117–124, 1983.
32. Brant-Zawadzki M.: Nuclear magnetic resonance imaging: The abnormal brain and spinal cord, in Newton T.H., Potts D.G. (eds.): *Modern Neuro-*

radiology. Vol. 2: *Advanced Imaging Techniques.* San Anselmo, Clavadel Press, 1983.

33. McGinnis B.D., Brady T.J., New P.F.J., et al.: Nuclear magnetic resonance (NMR) imaging of tumors in the posterior fossa. *J. Comput. Assist. Tomogr.* 7:575–584, 1983.

34. Randell C.P., Collins A.G., Young I.R., et al.: Nuclear magnetic resonance of posterior fossa tumors. *AJNR* 4:1027–1034, 1983.

35. Bydder G.M., Steiner R.E., Thomas D.J., et al.: Nuclear magnetic resonance imaging of the posterior fossa: 50 cases. *Clin. Radiol.* 34:173–188, 1983.

36. DeLaPaz R.L., Brady T.J., Buonanno F.S., et al.: Nuclear magnetic resonance (NMR) imaging of Arnold Chiari type I malformation with hydromyelia. *J. Comput. Assist. Tomogr.* 7:126–129, 1983.

37. Han J.S., Kaufman B., Alfidi R.J., et al.: Head trauma evaluated by magnetic resonance and computed tomography: A comparison. *Radiology* 150:71–77, 1984.

38. Modic M.T., Weinstein M.A., Pavlicek W., et al.: Nuclear magnetic resonance imaging of the spine. *Radiology* 148:757–762, 1983.

39. Han J.S. Kaufman B., El Yousef S.J., et al.: NMR imaging of the spine. *AJNR* 4:1151–1160, 1983.

40. Buonanno F.S., Pykett I.L., Brady T.J., et al.: Clinical relevance of two different nuclear magnetic resonance (NMR) approaches to imaging of low grade astrocytoma. *J. Comput. Assist. Tomogr.* 6:529–535, 1982.

41. Lawler G.A., Pennock J.M., Steiner R.E., et al.: Nuclear magnetic resonance (NMR) imaging in Wilson disease. *J. Comput. Assist. Tomogr.* 7:1–9, 1983.

42. Vermess M., Bernstein R.M., Bydder G.M., et al.: Nuclear magnetic resonance (NMR) imaging of the brain in systemic lupus erythematosus. *J. Comput. Assist. Tomogr.* 7:461–467, 1983.

43. Sipponen J.T., Kaste M., Ketonen L., et al.: Serial nuclear magnetic resonance (NMR) imaging in patients with cerebral infarction. *J. Comput. Assist. Tomogr.* 7:585–589, 1983.

44. Bryan R.N., Willcott M.R., Schneiders N.J., et al.: Nuclear magnetic resonance evaluation of stroke. *Radiology* 149:189–192, 1983.

45. Pykett I.L., Buonanno F.S., Brady T.J., et al.: True three dimensional nuclear magnetic resonance neuro-imaging in ischemic stroke: Correlation of NRM, x-ray, CT and pathology. *Stroke* 14:173–177, 1983.

46. Gamsu G., Webb W.R., Sheldon P., et al.: Nuclear magnetic resonance imaging of the thorax. *Radiology* 147:473–480, 1983.

47. Cohen A.M., Creviston S., Lipuma J.P., et al.: Nuclear magnetic resonance of the mediastinum and hili: Early impressions of its efficacy. *AJR* 141:1163–1169, 1983.

48. Axel L., Kressel H.Y., Thickman D., et al.: NMR imaging of the chest at 0.12T: Initial clinical experience with a resistive magnet. *AJR* 141:1157–1162, 1983.

49. Webb W.R., Gamsu G.: Chest, in Margulis A.R., Higgins C., Kaufman L., et al.: (eds.): *Clinical Magnetic Resonance Imaging.* San Francisco, Radiology Research and Education Foundation, 1983.

50. Ross R.J., Thompson J.S., Kim K., et al.: Nuclear magnetic resonance imaging and evaluation of human breast tissue: Preliminary clinical trials. *Radiology* 143:195–205, 1982.
51. Yousef S.J., Alfidi R.J., Duchesneau R.H., et al.: Initial experience with nuclear magnetic resonance imaging of the human breast. *J. Comput. Assist. Tomogr.* 7:215–218, 1983.
52. Lanzer P., Botvinick E.H., Schiller N.B., et al.: Cardiac imaging using gated magnetic resonance. *Radiology* 150:121–127, 1984.
53. Go R.T., MacIntyre W.J., Yeung H.N., et al.: Volume and planar gated cardiac magnetic resonance imaging: A correlative study of normal anatomy with thallium-201 SPECT and cadaver sections. *Radiology* 150:129–135, 1984.
54. Higgins C.B., et al.: Cardiovascular system, in Margulis A.R., Higgins C., Kaufman L., et al. (eds.): *Clinical Magnetic Resonance Imaging*. San Francisco, Radiology Research and Education Foundation, 1983.
55. Fletcher B.D., Jacobstein M.D., Nelson A.D., et al.: Gated magnetic resonance of congenital cardiac malformations, *Radiology* 150:137–140, 1984.
56. Herfkens R.J., Higgins C.B., Hricak H., et al.: Nuclear magnetic resonance imaging of the cardiovascular system: Normal and pathologic findings. *Radiology* 147:749–759, 1983.
57. Nunnally R.L., Bottomley P.A.: P-31NMR studies of myocardial ischemia and its response to drug therapies. *J. Comput. Assist. Tomogr.* 5:296, 1981.
58. Doyle F.H., Pennock J.M., Banks L.M., et al.: Nuclear magnetic resonance imaging of the liver: Initial experience. *AJR* 138:193–200, 1982.
59. Kressel H.Y., Axel L., Thickman D., et al.: NMR imaging of the abdomen at 0.12T: Initial clinical experience with a resistive magnet. *AJR* 150:1179–1186, 1983.
60. Moss A.A., Goldberg H.I., Stark D.D., et al.: Hepatic tumors: Magnetic resonance and CT appearance. *Radiology* 150:141–147, 1984.
61. Stark D.D., Bass N.M., Moss A.A., et al.: Nuclear magnetic resonance imaging of experimentally induced liver disease. *Radiology* 148:743–751, 1983.
62. Stark D.D., Goldberg H.I., Moss A.A., et al.: Chronic liver disease: Evaluation by magnetic resonance. *Radiology* 150:149–151, 1984.
63. Hricak H., Filly R.A., Margulis A.R., et al.: Work in progress: Magnetic resonance imaging of the gallbladder. *Radiology* 147:481–484, 1983.
64. Moon K.L., Hricak H., Margulis A.R., et al.: Nuclear magnetic resonance imaging characteristics of gallstones in vitro. *Radiology* 148:752–756, 1983.
65. Stark D.D., Moss A.A., Goldberg H.I., et al.: Magnetic resonance and CT of the normal and diseased pancreas: A comparative study. *Radiology* 150:153–162, 1984.
66. Moss A.A., et al.: Liver, gallbladder, alimentary tube, spleen, peritoneal cavity and pancreas, in Margulis A.R., et al. (eds.): *Clinical Magnetic Resonance Imaging,* San Francisco, Radiology Research and Education Foundation, 1983.
67. Moon K.L., Hricak H., Crooks L.E., et al.: Nuclear magnetic resonance

imaging of the adrenal gland: A preliminary report. *Radiology* 147:155–160, 1983.
68. Hricak H., Crooks L.E., Sheldon P., et al.: Nuclear magnetic resonance imaging of the kidney. *Radiology* 146:425–432, 1983.
69. Hricak H., Williams R.D., Moon K.L., et al.: Nuclear magnetic resonance imaging of the kidneys: Renal masses. *Radiology* 147:765–772, 1983.
70. Hricak H., Higgins C.B., Williams R.D.: Nuclear magnetic resonance imaging in retroperitoneal fibrosis. *AJR* 141:35–38, 1983.
71. Lipuma J.P., Bryan P.J., Cohen A.M., et al.: Renal transplant NMR, abstracted. Radiological Society of North America, 1983, Abstract No. 621.
72. Hricak H., Williams R.D., Spring D.B., et al.: Anatomy and pathology of the male pelvis by magnetic resonance imaging. *AJR* 141:1101–1110, 1983.
73. Hricak H., Alpers C., Crooks L.E., et al.: Nuclear magnetic resonance imaging of the female pelvis: Initial experience. *AJR* 141:1119–1128, 1983.
74. Bryan P.J., Butler H.E., Lipuma J.P., et al.: NMR scanning of the pelvis: Initial experience with a 0.3T system. *AJR* 141:1111–1118, 1983.
75. Brady T.J., Rosen B.R., Pykett I.L., et al.: NMR imaging of leg tumors. *Radiology* 149:181–187, 1983.
76. Moon K.L., Genant H.K., Helms C.A., et al.: Musculoskeletal applications of nuclear magnetic resonance. *Radiology* 147:161–171, 1983.
77. Fletcher B.D., Scoles P.V., Nelson A.D.: Osteomyelitis in children: Detection by magnetic resonance. *Radiology* 150:57–60, 1983.

New Approaches to Unusual Aneurysms

E. STANLEY CRAWFORD, M.D. AND
CARY L. STOWE, M.D.

From the Department of Surgery, Baylor College of Medicine and the Surgical Service of The Methodist Hospital, Houston, Texas.

MOST aortic aneurysms are limited in extent and involve one or more of the well-known anatomical segments of the aorta, such as the ascending aorta, transverse aortic arch, descending thoracic aorta, and infrarenal abdominal aorta. In some cases the disease may involve either the upper abdominal aorta, from which the visceral vessels arise, or the entire abdominal aorta. In other cases, both the descending thoracic and abdominal aorta may be affected. Techniques have been developed and are now being successfully employed in the treatment of most of these patients regardless of location and extent of disease.

An unusual manifestation of aortic aneurysmal disease is diffuse involvement of most or all of the aorta. This condition has been referred to by various terms, such as generalized aortic ectasia or "mega-aorta." Regardless of the terminology, the condition is truly aneurysmal in nature and its natural course terminates in rupture in most cases. Our approach to this problem in the past 4 years has been complete replacement of the involved aorta by combining total transverse aortic arch replacement with thoracoabdominal aortic resection in stages, the order of which is determined by clinical manifestations. Patients with large aneurysms of the ascending aorta and transverse aortic arch associated with aortic valve insufficiency or

67

coronary artery disease are treated first by ascending and transverse aortic arch replacement through an anterior incision; 6–8 weeks later the remaining aorta is replaced through a left posterolateral thoracoabdominal incision, as previously described.[5, 9] The order of aortic replacement is reversed in patients with large symptomatic thoracoabdominal components. To illustrate the effectiveness of graft replacement in these cases, this report relates our experience with total replacement of the aorta in ten patients, eight with medial degenerative disease and two with chronic aortic dissection and aneurysmal dilation of the false lumen.

Medial Degenerative Disease

Medial degenerative disease is the most common cause of thoracic aortic aneurysms, particularly when the ascending and transverse aortic arch is involved. The aneurysmal disease resulting from this abnormality is usually localized to a single aortic segment, but it may be the cause of diffuse involvement of the thoracic aorta and varying segments of abdominal aorta up to and including the entire aorta. Eight of our ten patients who required total aortic replacement had diffuse aneurysmal disease due to medial degeneration. Grossly, the diameter of the involved aorta, as determined by aortography, CT scanning, and examination at operation, was 3–10 times normal and varied from patient to patient, within each patient, and by the aortic segment under consideration. The aortic wall was of normal thickness and pliable with a texture similar to newly tanned leather. In general, the intima was smooth and grayish pink. Soft yellow patches of varying sizes representing intimal atheromatous deposits were frequently observed. These could be easily wiped away with gauze, leaving exposed media. The adventitial layer appeared normal or slightly fibrotic in some cases. Although the aortic wall appeared to be tough, it was frequently friable, requiring careful suturing and sometimes reinforcement with strips of Dacron and Teflon felt to prevent cutting of aortic tissue.

Microscopically, the adventitial and intimal layers of aorta in these patients were similar to those of patients of similar ages in whom the aorta was considered normal. The principal abnormal changes occurred in the medial layer and involved to varying degrees all regions from which biopsy specimens were obtained. Changes in elastic tissue and smooth muscle lamellae varied from fragmentation to total disappearance. There was abundant ground substance (acid mucopolysaccharide) between the elastic tissue fibers throughout the specimens (myxomatous or myxoid degeneration), with pools of this substance in areas of loss of normal media tissue (Erdheim's idiopathic cystic medial necrosis). Thus, changes observed in these cases were identical to those described in myxomatous and myxoid degeneration, Erdheim's cystic medial necrosis, Marfan's disease, and advanced aging. For this reason, we prefer the broader but more accurate term "medial degenerative disease" for this condition.

Clinical Features

Of the eight patients with diffuse degenerative medial disease involving the entire aorta, six (75%) were women and two (25%) were men, the reverse of the ratio reported in patients with aneurysmal disease of the abdominal aorta. Their ages ranged from 58 to 71 years (mean, age 65 years). Thus, the condition was seen primarily in women in the later years of life expectancy. Most of the women were heavy smokers, thin, and frail. The two men were in good muscular and nutritional condition. Associated disease was common in both men and women except as indicated. Moderately severe obstructive pulmonary disease with mild to moderate respiratory insufficiency affected four of the women (50%). Hypertension was present in five (63%), coronary artery disease in two, and occlusive vascular disease of the lower extremities in one patient. Aortic valve insufficiency, cardiomegaly, and impaired left ventricular function were present in three patients.

Clinical manifestations of aneurysm included chest pain in six (75%) and aortic diastolic murmurs in three (38%). Two patients were asymptomatic at presentation. Large mediastinal masses were evident in all patients on roentgenographic examination (Fig 1). The full extent of aneurysmal involvement was present at the time of first admission in all eight patients.

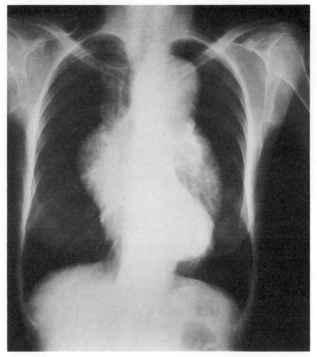

Fig 1.—The typical plain roentgenographic appearance of patients with diffuse aortic aneurysmal disease resulting from medial degeneration.

Chronic Aortic Dissection

Aortic dissection with late dilation of the false lumen is the second most common etiology of aneurysm in the thoracic aorta. Depending on the location, origin, and extent of dissection, late aneurysmal formation may be confined to the ascending aorta, transverse aortic arch, descending thoracic aorta, or, in cases of type I dissection, the entire aorta up to and including the iliac vessels. Two of our ten patients who required total aortic replacement had late aneurysmal formation secondary to chronic type I aortic dissections; one of these had Marfan's syndrome.

Examination of the involved aorta by CT scan, aortography, and at operation revealed diffuse aneurysmal dilation of the entire thoracic and abdominal aorta. The aneurysmal dilation of the false lumen was 2–3 times the size of the normal aorta and in both patients followed the usual course of aortic dissections—along the greater curvature of the ascending and transverse arch, the left posterolateral aspect of the descending thoracic aorta, and the right or left posterolateral aspect of the abdominal aorta into the right or left common iliac artery (Fig 2). There was moderate fibrosis in the walls of the false lumen due to chronicity of the disease but the wall thickness varied according to the degree of dilation in the various segments.

Clinical Features

Both patients who underwent total aortic replacement for chronic aortic dissection were men. One patient was 51 years old, while the second patient, with Marfan's disease, was only

Fig 2.—Patient with chronic type I aortic dissection complicated by aortic valvular insufficiency and fusiform aneurysm involving the entire aorta. **A,** drawing and aortogram done before operation showing massive aneurysmal dilation of the false lumen throughout the aorta. The aneurysmal dilation extends along the greater curvature of the ascending and transverse arch and the left posterolateral wall of descending and abdominal aorta, compressing the true lumen on the right (the route of dissection in 90% of cases). **B,** method of graft replacement of the aortic valve and ascending and transverse aortic arch in the first operation. **C,** drawing and aortogram made after second operation showing total replacement of the aorta with preservation of intercostal, visceral, and lumbar circulation. (Copyright 1983, Baylor College of Medicine. Reproduced by permission.)

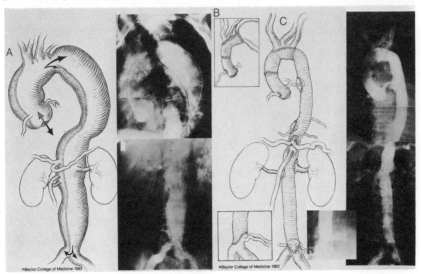

35. Systemic hypertension was the only other associated disease found and was present in both patients, but at admission was well controlled in the 120/80 mm Hg range with appropriate medications.

The 51-year-old man was seen 14 months after acute dissection and had done well on medical treatment until a recurrence of severe substernal and back pain suggested progression of the disease. The young patient with Marfan's disease was seen 39 months following acute dissection complicated by acute valvular insufficiency. At the time of the acute dissection, he was operated on in his hometown and was found to have a dissection superimposed on a fusiform aneurysm of the ascending aorta. He was treated by proximal ascending aortic transection, resuspension of the aortic valvular apparatus by oversewing the inner and outer layers of dissection proximally, and primary end-to-end anastomosis to the similarly oversewn distal ascending aortic segment. The dilated proximal ascending aorta was corsetted by completely enclosing it within a Dacron wrap. The patient recovered and did well until 39 months later, when cardiac evaluation revealed significant aortic insufficiency with "heart strain," an increase in size of the ascending aorta, and a large palpable abdominal aortic aneurysm.

Both patients were referred to us for evaluation. On admission, they were asymptomatic, but both demonstrated significant murmurs of aortic insufficiency. Aortograms revealed diffuse aneurysms of the entire aorta at the time of presentation.

Surgical Treatment

Treatment in these patients entailed replacement of the aneurysmal disease by graft with a staging operation to permit the best exposure and to limit the extent of operation to that best tolerated by the patient. Consequently, the ten patients underwent 21 operations during the period from Oct. 27, 1980 to Aug. 2, 1983. In general, operation was performed in two stages or by two anatomical approaches. The ascending aorta and transverse aortic arch were replaced in all ten patients at one operation. In nine patients the entire thoracic and abdominal aortas were replaced at a second operation. A single patient with mega-aorta due to medial degenerative disease required three operations for complete replacement of the aorta.

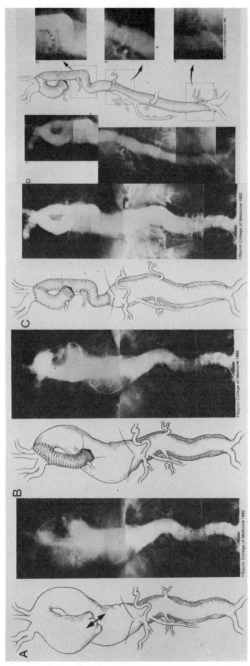

Fig 3.—Illustrations of treatment in a patient with aneurysm (**A**) involving the entire aorta with associated aortic valvular insufficiency. **B**, first operation on Aug. 20, 1980 consisted of total aortic arch replacement, including the aortic valve. **C**, the descending thoracic aortic segment was replaced Oct. 27, 1980. **D**, the abdominal segment subsequently enlarged, became painful, and was replaced on Dec. 29, 1981. Visceral vessels lumbar and intercostal arteries were reattached as shown in **D**. (Copyright 1982, Baylor College of Medicine. Reproduced by permission.)

Initially his entire thoracic aorta was replaced in two staged procedures. The abdominal aorta was saved because it was ectatic but not aneurysmal. The abdominal disease subsequently progressed to diffuse aneurysm, and it was resected and grafted electively at a third operation (Fig 3).

The operation for replacement of the ascending aorta and transverse aortic arch was performed through a midsternal incision employing heparinization, cardiopulmonary bypass, profound hypothermia, and circulatory arrest. The ascending aorta and transverse arch were replaced with a graft using inclusion technique, reattaching the brachiocephalic vessel origins directly to openings made in the side of the graft, as previously described.[7-11] Involvement of aortic root and aortic valve causing aortic valvular insufficiency was treated at the same operation in five patients by composite valve graft replacement, with the native coronary ostia directly reattached to openings made in the graft. Straight woven Dacron tube grafts were inserted by suture technique in the remaining five patients. Intraluminal grafts with extensions for future attachment of distal grafts have been inserted for total arch replacement in three additional patients with diffuse aneurysmal disease who are awaiting this second procedure, a technique originally described by Borst (Fig 4).[2] Femoral artery perfusion was used to induce hypothermia, but to prevent the development of cerebral emboli from distal aortic debris, perfusion during the warm-up period was done through sidearm grafts placed in the graft employed to replace the aortic arch (Fig 5).

The descending thoracic and abdominal aortic segments were replaced in ten patients without heparinization and without shunts through a left thoracoabdominal incision using inclusion technique and pharmacologic agents to control circulatory hemodynamics during aortic cross-clamping, as previously described.[3, 5] The proximal end of the graft was attached to the graft employed for arch replacement. The abdominal aortic segment was exposed retroperitoneally by reflecting the left colon, kidney, spleen, stomach, and body and tail of the pancreas upward and to the right. The origins of the visceral vessels were reattached directly to openings made in the graft. Intercostal and lumbar arteries were similarly reattached, when patent, in seven and four patients, respectively (see Figs 2 and 3).

The sequence of operations was determined by the clinical

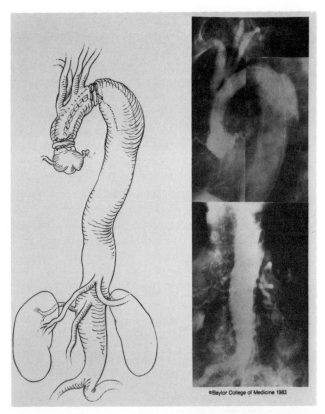

Fig 4.—Illustration of use of specially designed intraluminal graft for replacement of ascending and transverse aortic arch. The drawing and aortogram done after first operation, show that the specially designed intraluminal graft is in place and functioning. (Copyright 1983, Baylor College of Medicine. Reproduced by permission.)

manifestations and the size of the aneurysm in a particular aortic segment. The interval between operations was determined by the period of recovery from the first operation, the condition of the patient at the time of maximum recovery, and the progress of disease in the unreplaced aortic segments. The ascending aortic and arch segments of aorta were replaced as the primary operation in all ten patients to correct heart strain imposed by aortic valvular insufficiency in five and as the desired elective approach in five.

The interval between first and final operations varied from 27 days to 10 months, the usual interval being 3 months. Op-

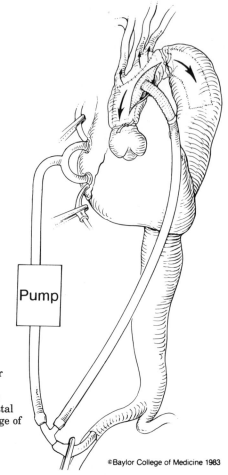

Fig 5.—Intraluminal graft with "elephant trunk extension" in place for future attachment of distal graft with proximal perfusion during warm-up to prevent cerebral embolization from distal disease. (Copyright 1983, Baylor College of Medicine. Reproduced by permission.)

©Baylor College of Medicine 1983

eration was delayed for 6 months in one patient to allow recovery from hepatitis.

Results

All ten patients survived graft replacement of their entire thoracic and abdominal aorta for diffuse aneurysmal disease. Three patients died during the follow-up period. One patient died 68 days postoperatively from sepsis and pulmonary failure following perforation of a colon diverticulum. Another patient was a small, debilitated woman with severe chronic obstructive pulmonary disease who died in the hospital 39 days following operation with pneumonia and pulmonary failure. The third death was in a patient with medial degenerative disease who died of unknown causes 26 months after operation, but she had a known history of atherosclerotic coronary artery disease. At this time, seven patients (70%) are alive.

No patients developed cerebral problems and only one patient developed neurologic complications in the lower extremities. This patient had total aortic replacement for chronic dissection. Two intercostal arteries were reattached to the graft at the midthoracic level and three intercostal arteries were attached just above the diaphragm. The last set of lumbar arteries were preserved by the technique demonstrated in Figure 2,C. The operation proceeded without complications, but postoperatively the patient had weakness of the right hip flexors and adductors and a neurogenic bladder. The patient was immediately started on physical therapy, and by discharge from the hospital 6 weeks later, he was walking with a walker and voiding by self-catheterization. At the last follow-up, 1 year from discharge, the patient's bladder function had completely recovered and he was walking unaided.

Discussion

Aneurysmal disease of the thoracic aorta is a serious condition because the actuarial 5-year survival of nontreated patients is only 13%, with most patients dying from ruptures. The disease is frequently multicentric, with other aortic segments being involved in more than 25% of cases.[1, 6, 12] In surgically treated cases in which the principal thoracic lesion is successfully replaced, one of the most common causes of both early and late death is rupture of a second aneurysm.[12] The clinical significance of these observations is the need for complete aortic examination for diagnosis and planned replacement of the associated aneurysmal disease to achieve maximum survival.[6]

One factor responsible for the higher incidence of diffuse aortic involvement with aneurysms of the thoracic aorta is the underlying etiology of the aneurysm. Medial degeneration is the most common cause of aneurysm of the ascending and transverse aortic arch and it diffusely involves the entire aortic media. The medial degeneration, as previously described, often involves the aorta diffusely in the elderly population, while it may be associated with multiple lesions in younger patients.[4] The diffuse nature of the disease can lead to total aortic aneurysm, as seen in our eight patients with mega-aorta.

Aortic dissections are probably a result of a medial degenerative disorder of the aortic wall potentiated by systemic hypertension. The location of the dissecting channel is in the outer half of the aortic media, and as a consequence, the outer wall of the false channel is very thin, making the wall of the false lumen susceptible to early rupture or aneurysmal formation. In 65% of patients, the dissection originates in the ascending aorta and extends distally to involve the entire aorta.[13] A large percentage of these patients die during the acute episode, and long-term follow-up of survivors indicates formation of aneurysm in the false lumen in 30% of patients within a period of 5 years, and death in 29% of untreated patients. Thus, chronic type I dissection and medial degenerative disease are the etiologies of aneurysms that ultimately require total aortic replacement.

There is no precedence for total aortic graft replacement, but techniques are available for this purpose. Total aortic arch replacement is being reported with a high incidence of survival in relatively large series of patients with aneurysmal disease limited to the aortic arch, and extensive graft replacement of thoracoabdominal aortic aneurysm is being reported also with success in over 90% of patients with aneurysm limited to this segment of the aorta.[3, 5, 7, 9] Therefore, it seemed logical for us to consider application of both of these procedures in stages for aneurysmal disease of the entire aorta. The rationale of treatment in these patients was, first, graft replacement of the life-threatening aortic segment, and second, replacement of the remaining segment at a second operation, either as required by the course of the disease or electively as permitted by the condition of the patient. We have now completed total aortic replacement in ten patients, and seven patients are still alive from 6 months to 3½ years since completion of treatment. A new concept of modality of therapy is suggested and its position in the overall treatment of aortic disease will be established by further application.

REFERENCES

1. Bickerstaff L.K., Pairolero P.C., Hollier L.H., et al.: Thoracic aortic aneurysms: A population-based study. *Surgery* 92:1103 1108, 1982.
2. Borst H.G., Walterbusch G., Schaps D.: Extensive aortic replacement using "elephant trunk" prosthesis. *Thorac. Cardiovasc. Surg.* 31:37–40, 1983.
3. Crawford E.S.: Thoraco-abdominal and abdominal aortic aneurysms involving renal, superior mesenteric, and celiac arteries. *Ann. Surg.* 179:763–772, 1974.
4. Crawford E.S.: Marfan's syndrome: Broad spectral surgical treatment cardiovascular manifestations. *Ann. Surg.* 198:487–505, 1983.
5. Crawford E.S., Cho G.C., Roehm J.O.F., Jr.: Thoraco-abdominal and abdominal aortic aneurysms involving celiac axis, superior mesenteric, and renal arteries, in Bergan J.J., Yao J.S.T. (eds.): *Surgery of the Aorta and its Body Branches.* New York, Grune & Stratton, 1979, pp. 145–169.
6. Crawford E.S., Cohen E.S.: Aortic aneurysm: A multifocal disease. *Arch. Surg.* 117:1393–1400, 1982.
7. Crawford E.S., Saleh S.A.: Transverse aortic arch aneurysm: Improved results of treatment employing new modifications of aortic reconstruction and hypothermic cerebral circulatory arrest. *Ann. Surg.* 194:180–199, 1981.
8. Crawford E.S., Snyder D.M.: Aneurysms of the thoracic aorta: Basic principles of surgical treatment. *Contemp. Surg.* 21:34–49, 1982.
9. Crawford E.S., Snyder D.M.: Treatment of aneurysms of the aortic arch: A progress report. *J. Thorac. Cardiovasc. Surg.* 85:237–246, 1983.
10. Crawford E.S., Stowe C.L., Crawford J.L., et al.: Total aortic replacement for chronic aortic dissection occurring in patients with and without Marfan's Syndrome. *Ann. Surg.* 199:358–359, 1984.
11. Crawford E.S., Stowe C.L., Crawford J.L., et al.: Aortic arch aneurysm: A sentinel of extensive aortic disease requiring subtotal and total aortic replacement. *Ann. Surg.,* to be published.
12. Crawford E.S., Walker H.S.J. III, Saleh S.A., et al.: Graft replacement aneurysm descending thoracic aorta: Results without bypass or shunting. *Surgery* 89:73–85, 1981.
13. Roberts W.C.: Pathology of arterial aneurysms, in Bergan J.J., Yao J.S.T. (eds.): *Aneurysms: Diagnosis and Treatment.* New York, Grune & Stratton, 1981, pp. 17–43.

Selective Variceal Decompression: Current Status and Recent Advances

J. MICHAEL HENDERSON, F.R.C.S. AND
W. DEAN WARREN, M.D.

*From the Joseph B. Whitehead Department of Surgery, Emory University
School of Medicine, Atlanta, Georgia*

THIS CHAPTER reviews the development, application, and evolution of selective variceal decompression since its introduction in the mid-1960s.[1] The basic concept of selective shunting—the control of bleeding from gastroesophageal varices while maintaining portal perfusion of the liver to preserve hepatic function—has been well documented. However, as data and experience have accumulated, lessons have been learned and modifications made in technique and patient management. In this chapter we outline these advances and present our current recommendations for selective variceal decompression.

The historical factors leading to the introduction of selective shunting can be summarized as follows:

1. The long-term results of portacaval shunts showed excellent control of bleeding but unacceptable mortality and morbidity secondary to hepatic failure and encephalopathy.[2-4]

2. Nonshunt devascularization procedures were accompanied by a very low incidence of portal-systemic encephalopathy but were unsatisfactory because of significant rebleeding.[5, 6]

3. Hemodynamic studies pinpointed maintenance of portal

81

0065-3411/84/0018-0081-0116-$04.00

venous perfusion and portal hypertension as critical in preserving hepatic function.[7-9]

Portal-systemic shunts, introduced in the 1940s, provided total decompression of portal hypertension and prevented death from recurrent variceal bleeding. It took controlled clinical trials, initially with prophylactic shunts[10-12] in the 1950s and then with therapeutic shunts[2-4, 13] in the 1950s and 1960s, to show the true picture. In individual studies no advantage in survival was ever shown in patients having total portal-systemic shunts compared to those having conventional medical management. Analysis of the four therapeutic studies[13] combined showed an advantage in survival to those who had surgery, but this was offset by incapacitating encephalopathy. Bleeding could be controlled by such shunts, but the mode of death was changed to hepatic failure.

Recognition that sudden total loss of portal venous perfusion was the main deleterious factor in precipitating liver failure following portacaval shunts led to the development of two alternative approaches. First, some workers attempted partial decompression of the portal hypertension with a variety of side-to-side shunts. Interposition mesocaval shunts, as popularized by Drapanas et al.,[14] were purported to decompress the varices yet maintain portal perfusion. This combination is untenable hemodynamically, and indeed the fallacy in the initial claims has been demonstrated by several groups[15, 16]: a mesocaval shunt which decompresses varices also decompresses the liver, with reversal of portal venous flow. The central splenorenal shunt, advocated by Linton et al.,[17] may initially permit some portal perfusion if it is not sufficiently large to totally decompress the portal system. However, with time, one of two things will happen: either the shunt will enlarge sufficiently to provide total decompression or it will thrombose, with maintenance of portal perfusion and return of gastroesophageal varices. The second alternative entailed nonshunt procedures,[5, 6] with extensive gastroesophageal devascularization but maintenance of portal hypertension and perfusion. These procedures preserved liver function but were followed by significant rebleeding.

Rationale for Selective Variceal Decompression

It was against this background that selective variceal decompression emerged in 1966.[1] The pathophysiologic rationale on which selective variceal decompression was based was totally different from the rationale underlying any previous shunt. The three fundamental goals of the distal splenorenal shunt (DSRS) were as follows:

1. Selective transsplenic decompression of gastroesophageal varices.

2. Maintenance of mesenteric and portal perfusion of the liver.

3. Maintenance of high intestinal venous pressure.

The DSRS is not a portal-systemic shunt. Portal hypertension is maintained, and it is only in the offending gastroesophageal segment that the varices are decompressed by the shunt. The first question to be answered was whether recurrent variceal bleeding could be controlled by such a selective shunt. If this could be achieved, the second and third goals, concerned with maintenance of hepatic function, become relevant. It was postulated that both the quantity and quality of blood flow delivered by the portal vein was integral to maximizing function in the already damaged liver. Could this be maintained and would it help maintain adequate hepatic function?

Scope of This Review

Assessment of the current status of any operative procedure depends on three types of information. First, there is the reported clinical experience of those using the procedure. Most of this is uncontrolled observation, usually presented by those who have had success with the procedure, which suggests the extent of its application. Second, there are controlled, prospective, randomized studies in which the new operation is compared with currently accepted operations. These studies provide an objective way of deciding the superiority of one type of procedure over another, but conclusions may be influenced by flaws in study design. Finally, when an operation purports to achieve specific aims, in this case maintain hepatic portal perfusion and function while decompressing varices, objective data must be presented in support of such claims.

The data which can be invoked to make these judgments now encompasses an enormous worldwide literature, with reports issuing from the United States, South America, Europe, Africa, Japan, and China. We will summarize this reported experience to assess which patients are being treated, and how successfully, by selective shunts.

The following section discusses the technical aspects and advances that relate to the DSRS. This prototype for selective variceal decompression is the shunt most widely used, but significant technical advances continue to be made which further implement and fulfill the original aims.

Method of the DSRS

Success of any operative method depends on correct preoperative evaluation and preparation, meticulous execution of all phases of the procedure, and optimal postoperative care. Inevitably with experience each of these phases evolve over time, and in this section we will outline the method as it has evolved at Emory University after 450 DSRS procedures.

PREOPERATIVE ASSESSMENT AND PREPARATION

Ideally, DSRS is carried out in the stable cirrhotic or noncirrhotic patient with variceal bleeding as an elective operation. The results of any shunt procedure will always be best in such populations, but the ideal situation must be qualified in two respects. First, the DSRS should not be denied to either the patient who continues to bleed or the patient who never achieves good results on liver function tests (Child's Class C); the notion that DSRS should only be done in Child's Class A or B patients and as an elective procedure should be laid to rest. Second, while the ideal patient has not changed, there have been dramatic improvements in the means of achieving that ideal over the past 10 years. Better control of acute bleeding with pitressin,[18] endoscopic sclerosis,[19, 20] and transhepatic embolization buy time to evaluate patients and optimize their condition. Nutritional management, with better understanding of the specific problems of cirrhosis and improved methods for control of ascites and coagulation abnormalities, now help in achieving the ideal more frequently. In our experience, 70% of patients admitted with acute bleeding can be brought to this stage.

There are three main steps in the essential preoperative evaluation of patients for DSRS, as follows.

1. Biochemical and hematologic tests. Bilirubin and albumin levels and prothrombin time prolongation remain good indicators of the severity of liver damage, provided they are interpreted in light of significant clinical events—for example, the time relationship to the acute bleeding episode. Liver enzyme and immunoglobulin levels and hepatitis antigen-antibody status should be measured to clarify the type and status of the liver disease. Renal function, particularly in the patient with ascites, should be assessed from the blood ureanitrogen (BUN) level, creatinine level, and creatinine clearance value.

2. Liver biopsy. Biochemical assessment permits classification of liver disease to a certain point, but morphological information, obtained from a percutaneous needle biopsy specimen establishes the diagnosis and can be used to assess the activity of the underlying chronic liver disease that led to cirrhosis.[21] More than mild necroinflammatory disease, polymorphonuclear infiltrate, and new collagen formation point to active liver disease, which is best treated prior to operation if time permits. Management of chronic active hepatitis with steroids, abstinence in alcoholic hepatitis, and appropriate nutritional support will help stabilize the liver process and reduce operative risks.

3. Visceral panangiography.[22] Superior mesenteric and splenic arterial studies are carried through their venous phase to visualize portal venous perfusion, splenic vein anatomy, and the origin, size, and direction of significant collateral veins. Definition of the latter requires emphasis, as they must be divided for adequate portal azygous disconnection. Venous catheterization measures wedged hepatic vein pressure, and wedge injection of contrast is the best way of defining reversal of portal venous flow. In addition, left renal vein anatomy is examined and the pressure measured. This examination is particularly valuable, as up to 20% of left renal veins are anomalous, and while an anomalous vein does not preclude a DSRS, it is preferable to know of the anomaly prior to operation.

Quantitative Liver Tests

The DSRS aims to preserve hepatic function, and assessment is most accurately done with quantitative tests. We have published details of the quantitative assessment that all shunt patients receive prior to and serially after DSRS at Emory University.[23] Measurement of liver and spleen size, effective liver blood flow, hepatocyte function, and basic nitrogen metabolism allows meaningful assessment of liver function changes after DSRS.

PERIOPERATIVE MANAGEMENT

The basic principles of good preoperative, intraoperative, and postoperative care apply to this group of patients, but several points specific to the cirrhotic patient require emphasis.

Fluid and Electrolytes

Sodium restriction is important at all stages of management because of the propensity of cirrhotic patients to form ascites. Dietary intake of sodium is restricted to 2 gm/day prior to and following surgery. No sodium containing intravenous crystalloid is used prior to, during, or after surgery. Effective plasma and blood volume is maintained with blood, fresh frozen plasma, or 5% albumin. The ascitic response in patients undergoing selective shunt, who maintain portal hypertension, can be minimized by strict adherence to such a regimen. The increased aldosterone response of cirrhotics can be blocked with spironolactone, which is given preoperatively and postoperatively; careful plasma and urine electrolyte monitoring is mandatory after surgery to avoid hyponatremia or hyperkalemia. A urine sodium to potassium ratio greater than 1 indicates adequate blockade of sodium resorption.

The final specific fluid problem seen after DSRS is chylous ascites. This occurs in 10%–20% of patients in the early postoperative period and is secondary to division of lymphatics around the mesenteric vessels at the time of dissection of the left renal vein. Dietary fat restriction to 30 gm/day is advised for 6–8 weeks after DSRS operation and has minimized this complication.

Medications

Diuretics should be used with caution. Spironolactone, used as described above, is important in the prevention and control of ascites; other diuretics should only be used when they are specifically indicated.

Cimetidine is given intravenously preoperatively, perioperatively, and early postoperatively to reduce gastric acid secretion and is followed by oral ranitidine. This combination has reduced postoperative gastritis bleeding and should be continued for 6 weeks.

Prophylactic antibiotic coverage should be given perioperatively. A cephalosporin given 2 hours preoperatively, every 2 hours intraoperatively, and with the final dose in the recovery room is a suitable regimen.

Dexamethasone (40 mg intravenously) is given by us 6 hours prior to operation and every 6 hours for 24 hours after operation. Preloading of hepatocytes with steroids in animals protects them from shock and is, we believe, beneficial for the occasional patient with high blood loss.

POSTOPERATIVE RADIOLOGIC STUDY

Evaluation prior to discharge at 7–10 days should routinely include angiography to demonstrate shunt patency and portal flow. When patent, the shunt is readily visualized on venous phase splenic artery study, but when there is doubt as to patency or a question of physiologic obstruction, the shunt should be catheterized for pressure studies. An unexpected problem at this time can be surgically corrected, whereas reexploration of a previously dissected splenic vein at a later time becomes increasingly difficult. Renal vein hypertension with documented shunt patency in the early postoperative period may result in inadequate early variceal decompression and should be managed expectantly. Resolution of retroperitoneal edema and the development of renal vein collaterals over 4–6 weeks will ultimately allow full decompression. Early postshunt bleeding (seen in up to 10% of patients) suggests this diagnosis. Provided shunt patency is demonstrated angiographically, nonoperative management is indicated.

THE OPERATION

A step-by-step description of the method for DSRS has recently been reviewed,[24] and this paper is essential reading for any surgeon performing DSRS operations. The major points of emphasis are as follows:

1. Mobilization of the pancreas. The most common error made in performing DSRS operation is failure to mobilize the

pancreas, which in turn leads to improper and incomplete dissection of the splenic vein.

2. Dissection of the splenic vein. The salient points here are (1) do the dissection of the vein on the vein; (2) dissect the posterior surface of the splenic vein before dissecting the anterior surface; (3) gain control of the splenic vein-portal vein junction; (4) dissection of the splenic vein must be sufficient to achieve a normal anatomical (i.e., nonkinked) relationship for anastomosis.

3. The anastomosis. This must be constructed without tension, but the redundant vein must be excised to avoid kinking. Usually the anastomosis is placed just anterior to the ligated adrenal vein orifice on the left renal vein. Although the posterior wall is completed with a continuous suture, we believe it is important to interrupt the anterior row sutures. Continuous suture to both rows leads to a purse string effect, which may narrow the anastomosis and preclude enlargement of the orifice. This latter may occur spontaneously with splenic vein enlargement or be performed angiographically by balloon dilation for stenosis.[25]

4. Coronary disconnection. Separation of the high-pressure portomesenteric axis from the low-pressure gastrosplenic compartment is an important component of selective shunts. This is one of the major areas of advance and is discussed in more detail below.

Recent Advances

The DSRS has evolved considerably since its introduction 17 years ago. While the originally stated aims of variceal decompression and maintenance of portal hypertension and portal venous flow remain unchanged, the technical means of achieving these ends have changed. Areas of recent advances in the operative method are in approach to emergency decompression, new methods for portosplenic disconnection, and the use of alternative selective shunts.

Splenocaval Shunt

Selective variceal decompression by direct splenocaval anastomosis has the theoretical advantage of bypassing the left renal vein, which may act as a significant obstruction to splenic outflow early after a conventional DSRS operation.[26]

Renal vein hypertension must be avoided in the patient having emergency shunting; early complete variceal decompression is mandatory to stop the bleeding. The contributors to renal vein outflow obstruction are a large increase in flow from the spleen and compression of the vein by the superior mesenteric artery and accompanying lymphatics. In cirrhosis the lymphatics may be greatly engorged and distended, and dissection of the left renal vein tends to exacerbate this process. Left renal vein hypertension (> 10 mm Hg gradient from the left renal vein to cava) occurs in approximately 20% of conventional DSRS operations, is a major consideration in emergency shunts, and is the factor that has led to the evolution of direct splenocaval shunts.

The technical aspects of splenocaval shunt construction are not strikingly different from the standard DSRS operation. Sufficient splenic vein must be mobilized from the pancreas; a larger spleen and tortuous vein facilitate this phase. The splenic vein is usually long enough to reach the cava unless the spleen is small and there is a direct, short splenic vein. Dissection of the inferior vena cava requires taking down the ligament of Treitz and mobilizing the fourth part of the duodenum. The cava is then approached anterior to the aorta, posterior to the superior mesenteric artery, and inferior to the left renal vein. The latter may act as a guide to the cava. Approximately 6–8 cm of infrarenal cava is mobilized, sufficient for a side clamp to be placed. A 0.5–1-cm button is excised from the cava and the anastomosis is fashioned as for a conventional DSRS.

Preliminary evaluation of this method has shown good control of bleeding and a less than 5 mm Hg pressure gradient from the splenic vein to inferior vena cava at 7–10 days after shunt. Further evaluation is required to fully define this new approach, which appears to be of particular value when early variceal decompression is required.

Splenopancreatic Disconnection

The aim of this new technical component to selective transsplenic variceal decompression is to interrupt the collateral venous pathways that develop, over time, from the high-pressure portal system to the low-pressure splenic system after DSRS.[27]

Why is this modification required? Four observations in patients following conventional DSRS led to the evolution and current evaluation of this new approach:

1. Patients with retained portal venous perfusion after DSRS have significantly better liver function than those who lose perfusion.[28]

2. Liver volume falls significantly after a DSRS operation[23, 29] whether or not portal perfusion is maintained.

3. Liver volume is better maintained in an equivalent group of patients with cirrhosis managed by longitudinal endoscopic sclerotherapy.

4. Transpancreatic venous pathways are a major route of collateral development to the splenic vein still embedded in the pancreas after conventional DSRS.

Relevant data pertaining to these observations are presented in more detail later. For now, suffice it to say that quantitative hemodynamic and hepatic function data emphasize the importance of maintaining portal perfusion and preventing formation of venous collateral paths to the shunt. An additional question raised by the quantitative data is why significant reduction in liver volume occurs after DSRS despite the maintenance of portal perfusion in 60% of patients. The importance of pancreatic hormones in prevention of hepatic atrophy has been well documented[30]: the "pancreatic siphon" (Fig 1), discussed in more detail below, progressively deprives the liver of insulin and glucagon as large transpancreatic collaterals develop to the shunt. Splenopancreatic disconnection (Fig 2) aims to reduce this siphon effect and better maintain portal perfusion.

Technically, the splenopancreatic disconnection involves the same basic approach to the splenic vein on the posterior surface of the pancreas, with the following additions:

1. The splenocolic ligament and splenic flexure should be taken down to allow better exposure and access for complete mobilization of the pancreas, with the additional benefit of ligating potential collateral pathways.

2. The body and tail of the pancreas must be fully mobilized right into the splenic hilus.

3. The splenic vein must be dissected totally free of the pancreas up to its bifurcation at the splenic hilus.

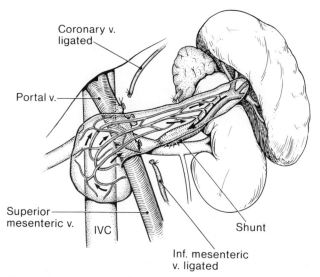

Fig 1.—The pancreatic siphon with a conventional DSRS. Pancreatic veins connect the high-pressure portal venous system to the low-pressure intrapancreatic splenic vein. Enlargement of these pathways occurs over time with drainage of pancreatic hormones to the systemic circulation. (From *Annals of Surgery*, Volume 199, 1984. Reproduced by permission.)

4. The pancreas should be retained within the portal hypertensive drainage bed of the mesenteric/hepatic axis for delivery of hepatotropic factors.

This new approach, while theoretically appealing, is still in its developmental stage. Dissection of the splenic vein at the hilus is fraught with danger, as a single mistake at this point can render the vein unusable for shunt. Critical evaluation with respect to liver size and function and the development of portaprival collaterals is under way.

Alternative Methods of Selective Shunts

The DSRS has become the primary operation for selective variceal decompression worldwide, but under certain circumstances an alternative approach may be required. The Japanese have demonstrated the feasibility of the coronary caval shunt,[31] but technical difficulties and lower patency rates have limited its application. We recently reviewed our experience with selective shunts in patients who had prior splenectomy or splenic vein thrombosis concurrently.[27] Our experience suggests the following: (1) splenectomy should not be done for thrombocytopenia associated with portal hypertension; (2) splenectomy does not preclude a selective shunt; and (3) full preoperative angiography, plus operative exploration for shuntable veins, should be undertaken in these patients.

Figure 3 illustrates diagrammatically the potential veins which may be used for selective shunt. We believe that the optimum vessel is the splenic vein, but low-pressure variceal drainage can be achieved through any for the four named pathways in the figure, either singly or in combination, while high-pressure mesenteric/portal venous flow is maintained to the liver.

Results

The current status of selective variceal decompression will be reviewed from the reported experience of nonrandomized series

Fig 2.—Splenopancreatic disconnection. Complete separation of the splenic vein from the pancreas interrupts the pancreatic collateral pathways. This permits both greater selectivity of variceal decompression and maintenance of pancreatic venous drainage to the portal system. (From Ann. Surg., Volume 199, 1984. Reproduced by permission.)

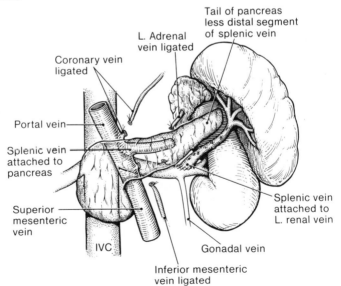

Tail of pancreas
less distal segment
of splenic vein

L. Adrenal
vein ligated

Coronary vein
ligated

Portal vein

Splenic vein
attached to
pancreas

Superior
mesenteric
vein

IVC

Splenic vein
attached to
L. renal vein

Gonadal vein

Inferior mesenteric
vein ligated

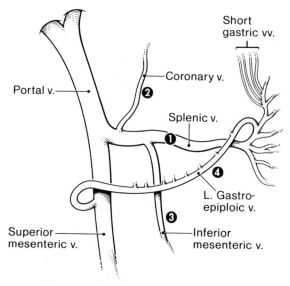

Fig 3.—The potential venous drainage pathways which may be used for selective variceal decompression *(1–4)*. Shunting may use these singly or in combination, with the high-pressure mesenteric/portal venous flow maintained to the liver. (From Ann Surg, Volume 199, 1984. Reproduced by permission.)

as well as prospective randomized clinical trials. This experience has recently been reviewed,[32] but we shall update it to the end of 1983 and summarize.

NONRANDOMIZED RESULTS WITH DSRS

The overall results in reported experiences fall into two distinct groups, with results achieved in North America differing in many respects from those achieved elsewhere. Diseases, diagnosis, management, and socioeconomic conditions vary enormously, so results must be interpreted in light of the best available option in any center at a given time.

North America

Reported experiences with DSRS are available from over ten centers in the United States.[33–44] The series include from 15 to 348 patients, with follow-up lasting from 6 months to 10 years. Of the total 620 patients, 60% had alcoholic cirrhosis and 40%

had a nonalcoholic etiology for portal hypertension, and 15% of the patients were in Child's class C. Certain common features emerge from these reports, such as operative mortality, survival, encephalopathy, and ascites, and most studies emphasize some other specific point, such as hemodynamics, hypersplenism, patency, or function. The salient features are reviewed below.

OPERATIVE MORTALITY.—The reported experience of the past 10 years shows an overall operative mortality of less than 6% (range, 1%–16%). This mortality, while primarily for elective operations, has included an increasing number of patients in Child's class C, and in our experience an increasing proportion of patients having shunt operation on an emergency basis. The mortality indicates that DSRS operation can now be performed in many centers with an acceptable operative mortality. Improvement and clarification of technique no longer limit DSRS to an operation performed by a few select surgeons.

SURVIVAL.—The length of follow-up in the reported series is variable, but analysis of those reporting at least 3 years' follow-up indicates a 70%–75% overall survival at 3 years and a 58% survival at 5 years. These figures, however, bear slightly closer scrutiny. Examination of the largest reported series from Emory University[33] shows two survival patterns after DSRS which are distinctly different from total shunt experience: first, survival patterns in patients in Child's classes A and B are virtually identical—63% at 5 years—and parallel the survival pattern seen historically in Child's class A patients following total shunts; second, nonalcoholics have significantly better survival than alcoholics (70% vs. 40% at 5 years). the nonalcoholic population in this series included many patients with chronic active hepatitis requiring steroid and/or Imuran therapy, not exclusively stable posthepatic cirrhotics. This parallels the experience of Zeppa et al. at Miami University,[34] who first showed the significantly improved survival in nonalcoholics. Their further analysis shows that the greatest contributor to late mortality in these patients is continuing active liver disease.[45] Martin et al.[36] also emphasizes an improvement in survival in the nonalcoholic population.

To what extent is the alcoholic patient's poorer survival related to continued alcohol intake? We have not been able to confirm the association,[29] but Zeppa et al. are on record as stating that alcohol consumption is an important determinant of survival.[45] Quantitative evaluation of these populations, as discussed below, may provide a key to the difference in survival between alcoholic and nonalcoholic patients.

ENCEPHALOPATHY.—Encephalopathy is a spectrum disorder ranging from coma, through the clinical syndrome of disorientation and asterixis, to the subclinical neuropsychological impairment which may be detected with psychometric testing and/or electroencephalography. The severe end of this spectrum is obviously catastrophic. Increasing attention is now being focused on the more subtle changes of the subclinical syndrome, as this may alter the patient's life-style. Management of the patient with cirrhosis who has bled from varices should extend beyond control of the bleeding to maintaining liver function and minimizing encephalopathy.

In uncontrolled studies the incidence of clinical encephalopathy is approximately 5% (range, 0–18%). No one has carefully assessed this complication in detail, probably because of the inherent difficulties of defining encephalopathy with its precipitating factors. This incidence is significantly lower after DSRS than after total portal decompression. Assessment of the available data suggests that encephalopathy seen in patients with total portal-systemic shunts is more likely to be severe, spontaneous, and incapacitating. The optimum management of encephalopathy should focus on prevention, and the significantly lower incidence and severity following DSRS is a logical first step in this management.

ASCITES.—The incidence of postshunt ascites occurring at a clinically detectable level ranges from 10% to 56%. This is usually transient and can be managed by salt restriction and diuretics; we have had to place LeVeen valves in only six patients (1.7%). If intractable ascites develops after DSRS operation and placement of a LeVeen valve becomes necessary, the valve placement should be delayed for 6 weeks, if possible. Preoperative ascites was initially considered a contraindication to DSRS because portal hypertension is maintained and numerous retroperitoneal lymphatics are divided. In 1984 it is only in the patient with truly intractable ascites preoperatively that DSRS is contraindicated.

HYPERSPLENISM.—The effect of DSRS on hypersplenism has been studied by several groups. Four of these report significant improvement in thrombocytopenia and leukopenia following DSRS. Analysis of our own data[27] defined a group of 33 patients with a platelet count below 50,000/cu mm. Splenic decompression resulted in significant ($P < .01$) improvement in the platelet count at 1 week, 6 months, and 1–3 years. There was no increased operative risk in this group, in whom variceal bleeding was successfully controlled. In addition, quantitative data have shown that spleen volume falls significantly after DSRS.

SHUNT PATENCY.—Postshunt angiography, performed in 30%–100% of patients in these series, demonstrated shunt patency in more than 90% of cases prior to hospital discharge. Is patency maintained? The only published data on long-term patency[46] indicate that late occlusion is rare, but shunt stenosis with physiologic obstruction has been documented.[25]

The high patency rate results from the direct vein-to-vein anastomosis and the high-flow "end shunt" of the splenic outflow tract. This patency also directly parallels the low incidence of rebleeding ($< 7\%$) after DSRS.

PORTAL VEIN THROMBOSIS.—The results of DSRS in patients with portal hypertension and variceal bleeding secondary to portal vein thrombosis warrant comment. Restoration of portal flow to a noncirrhotic liver by collaterals following portal vein occlusion was observed by Pavlov in 1893.[47] This was long ignored and the tacit assumption was made that portal vein thrombosis equated with no portal venous perfusion; therefore it was also assumed that a total portalsystemic shunt (usually mesocaval or central splenorenal) was the treatment of choice for variceal bleeding in such patients. However, in 1973 Voorhees et al. first showed that encephalopathy could indeed follow portalsystemic shunts in children.[48] This syndrome was different from the classic encephalopathy seen in cirrhotic patients and was manifested by behavioral changes and psychiatric abnormalities. The time scale in the development of neuropsychological impairment was also lengthened, presumably because the initially normal liver can compensate for total venous deprivation longer than a cirrhotic liver. Development of florid, protein-induced encephalopathy has been described 20 years after construction of a total shunt for portal vein thrombosis in a patient with an initially normal liver. Occlusion of the shunt with restoration of portal venous perfusion cleared the encephalopathy.[49]

Selective variceal decompression in this group of patients followed redocumentation that the high-pressure obstructed mesenteric system develops collaterals to the normal liver following portal vein thrombosis. The low pressure of the normal liver makes selective variceal decompression more favorable in this group than in cirrhotic patients because in the long term, the high-pressure mesenteric system collateralizes to the liver as readily as to the shunt.

The reported experience of DSRS in patients with portal vein thrombosis is relatively small,[49–51] with the common findings of technical feasibility and control of bleeding. Follow-up at this time is too short to make definitive statements concerning encephalopathy status, but early studies show maintenance of portal perfusion, liver size, and quantitative hepatocyte function.

Worldwide Experience

The DSRS has now undergone widespread trials in the management of variceal bleeding in many centers and in many patient populations with different etiologies for portal hypertension. All major European countries have reported on its use in cirrhotic patients. Increasingly from South America, Africa, and the Far East there have been reports on patients with schistosomiasis, in addition to patients with cirrhosis. These data must be assessed in light of what constituted standard therapy prior to selective shunting. We shall evaluate this experience based on the European experience and the data reported on schistosomiasis.

CIRRHOSIS.—The European experience encompasses nine countries with a combined reported total of 306 patients.[52–63] Sixty percent were alcoholic cirrhotics and 40% had nonalcoholic liver disease. The preoperative definition of the patients shunted indicate that 44% were in Child's class A, 47% were in Child's class B, and only 9% were in Child's class C: good to moderate risk patients are being selectively shunted. The operative mortality is 9% overall and is comparable to or lower than the mortality following other operative methods in such patients. Long-term survival is difficult to assess from the reported experience: some reports provide no follow-up data and in other series follow-up may be limited. Assessment at 3–5 years indicates a 45%–78% survival with a mean of approximately 60%. Many of these reports comment on the improved life-style or return to work following shunt. Encephalopathy does occur after DSRS but significantly less frequently and in less incapacitating form than after a total shunt in most series. Vang et al.[55] have clearly demonstrated that encephalopathy occurs earlier if there is no portal azygos disconnection.

SCHISTOSOMIASIS.—The commonest cause of portal hypertension and variceal bleeding worldwide is hepatosplenic schistosomiasis. Much of the available published data related to this problem are in the non-English-language literature. In 1978 Silvano Raia, from Sao Paulo, Brazil, published a comprehensive review of surgical methods for management of schistosomal portal hypertension.[64] The points that differentiate this condition from posthepatitic or alcoholic cirrhosis are the following: first, liver function is normal in the majority of patients; second, total portal venous diversion will flood the lungs with schistosomes; and third, encephalopathy is devastating and catastrophic after total shunts in these patients. Because of the high morbidity, total shunts were abandoned earlier in this population than in cirrhotic patients, and extensive non-shunt devascularization procedures were undertaken. While the advantage of the nonshunt procedures is avoidance of hepatic encephalopathy and liver failure, the disadvantages are significant rebleeding and the need for reoperation for bleeding in a large number of patients.

In the past 5 years reports of DSRS operation in patients with hepatosplenic schistosomiasis have emanated from Brazil,[64] Egypt,[65] and Puerto Rico.[66] The overall operative mortality achieved by these groups is 8%, with a high shunt patency rate and low incidence of rebleeding. At this time the low incidence of encephalopathy compares favorably with other reported experience.

Machado et al.,[66] in a review of their early experience with DSRS in this population, cited the following reasons for selective shunting in patients with schistosomiasis:

1. Liver function is usually excellent.
2. Ascites is an infrequent problem.
3. Severe or moderate hypersplenism improves after operation.
4. A large spleen is not a contraindication to DSRS.
5. The splenic vein is easier to dissect than in patients with cirrhosis.
6. The large short gastric veins provide an efficient decompressive route.

PROSPECTIVE RANDOMIZED STUDIES

In no field of medical clinical research is a prospective randomized study more difficult to implement than in the evaluation of a new surgical procedure. Yet surgeons must accept the challenge of evaluating new procedures against the accepted operation as an integral step in deciding whether or not it is superior. The specific problems facing the surgeon are several. The surgeon must master the new procedure to the extent that he is as technically competent with it as with the accepted standard. Once patients have been randomly assigned to an operative procedure (which should be at the time of surgery) and that procedure has been performed, the option to "cross over" therapy is lost. Finally, it takes longer, and is more difficult, to enter a large number of patients into a surgical treatment study than into a drug therapy study.

In this era of controlled clinical trials it is important that such studies be done, but it is equally important that they be interpreted in the light of overall experience, which may unmask factors lost within the limitations of such studies. Six prospective randomized clinical trials comparing DSRS with a variety of total portal-systemic shunts have been reported to date.[28, 67-72] Patients with cirrhosis and variceal bleeding were stabilized, evaluated for suitability for shunt, randomized, and underwent shunting as an elective operation. In one study patients were randomly assigned at the time of bleeding; in all other studies they were randomly assigned to a procedure just prior to operation.

The mortality figures for both DSRS and total shunts in these studies are presented in Table 1. Operative mortality has fluctuated between series, but when series are combined it is 10.6% for DSRS and 10.4% for total shunts. The late mortality has not been significantly different between the two shunt types in any study at any time. The time of reporting varies from 6 months to 10 years after operation, and results must be interpreted in light of the variance. However, in prospective randomized series, comparative survival is always meaningful in an ongoing series, and the combined survival of 69% at last reporting for DSRS was not significantly different from the 65% survival in patients with total shunts.

Why are these randomized studies at variance with the un-

TABLE 1.—SUMMARY OF SIX PROSPECTIVE RANDOMIZED STUDIES COMPARING DSRS WITH TOTAL PORTAL-SYSTEMIC SHUNTS

SHUNT	ETIOLOGY		OPERATIVE MORTALITY (%)	LATE* MORTALITY (%)	ENCEPHALOPATHY (%)	SHUNT OCCLUSION (%)
	Alc.	Nonalc.				
DSRS (N-132)	114	18	10.6	31	14	8.2
Total shunt (N-135)	108	27	10.4	35	36	9.7

*Length of follow-up, 6 months to 10 years.

controlled reported experience of improved survival after DSRS?

The majority of patients—83%—entered into these studies had alcoholic cirrhosis (see Table 1). The choice of this study population, which is markedly different from the nonrandomized experience, largely reflects the type of institution most likely to perform a randomized study and probably has significant bearing on the outcome of these studies. The nonrandomized experience from Miami University[34] and Emory University[33] has shown significantly improved survival in nonalcoholics compared to alcoholics after DSRS, a finding not seen following total shunts. It is of note that in our randomized group, six of the eight nonalcoholic patients that underwent DSRS operation are still alive, while only two of the seven given a total shunt are alive at a mean of 7.5 years. The randomized studies show no significant improvement in survival following DSRS in a predominantly alcoholic cirrhotic population.

The different types of total shunts performed in the combined studies (47% portacaval, 37% interposition H-graft, 16% central splenorenal) may have some influence on the results. The large number of interposition (Dacron) H-graft shunts reflects the climate of opinion in the early 1970s, when many of these studies were initiated: it was believed this was the best available total shunt at that time. This, however, proved to be wrong, as progressive thrombosis with time has been reported by several authors.[16, 73] Shunt occlusion leads to restoration of portal hypertension and portal perfusion, with the risk of further bleeding, but clearing of encephalopathy. Similarly, the central splenorenal shunt has been shown historically to be followed by a high incidence of thrombosis.[74] In the combined randomized experience, less than half of the total shunt group had a portacaval shunt—the only total shunt with *proved* long-term patency. This divergence in choices of total shunts will undoubtedly influence the final outcome of these studies. In our own experience, the H-grafts in six of the 13 survivors of total shunts have thrombosed at 7.5 years. In four of these portal perfusion was restored, and two had rebleeding from varices and required sclerotherapy. In contrast, all 12 surviving DSRS patients studied at a mean of 7.5 years after operation had patent shunts.[46] It is important to know the shunt status in the long-term follow-up of these patients, and we strongly urge such documentation in these studies.

Encephalopathy has occurred less frequently in the DSRS group in all studies except one. Encephalopathy has been judged and evaluated on a clinical basis and in many cases has been precipitated by bleeding, sepsis, or azotemia. The incidence of 36% overall in the total shunt experience represents the general reported level with total portal-systemic shunting, approximately half having severe impairment. The overall 14% incidence after DSRS includes predominantly mild precipitated encephalopathy. Severe spontaneous encephalopathy in these patients requires full evaluation and treatment as suggested by Conn et al.[71] An inadequate portal-azygos disconnection can be remedied.

In summary, these prospective randomized clinical trials to date have shown no significant improvement in survival from variceal bleeding in alcoholic cirrhotic patients managed by DSRS compared to those given a total shunt. The incidence of severe encephalopathy is lower following DSRS, and the control of bleeding is similar. Extrapolation of these data to all groups of patients with portal hypertension and variceal bleeding is not justified, as large nonrandomized studies have shown that long-term survival is related to disease etiology.

QUANTITATIVE DATA

This section evaluates data on the hemodynamic and hepatic function changes associated with DSRS. This area is exceedingly complex because of the diverse etiologies leading to the portal hypertension, which in their own right alter hemodynamics and function and are now also affected by the shunt. For example, cirrhosis is a spectrum disorder ranging from virtually normal hepatic size, function, and hemodynamics at one extreme, to the small liver with no hepatocyte reserve and loss of portal perfusion at the other extreme. This end stage may be approached through predominant loss of any of these three components, but is usually a combination of all in differing proportions. Evaluation of how far any shunt procedure affects the natural history of this process requires a clear understanding of the pathophysiology. Some of the data presented below begins to approach these questions.

Hemodynamics

ANGIOGRAPHY.[22]—Evaluation of portal venous hemodynamics by angiography is complex and open to significant mechanical and pharmacologic manipulation by the radiologist. However, standardized visceral artery angiography carried through to the venous phase and supplemented at times by splenoportography or direct transhepatic venous portography has evolved as the most widely implemented method of study of portal perfusion and venous anatomy. While it cannot be considered quantitative, angiography allows general assessment of whether prograde portal perfusion is good, moderate, poor, or lost. In addition, it permits mapping of portaprival collateral pathways. What data have been accumulated on portal perfusion following DSRS?

Early postshunt angiography—within the first month—has shown continuing portal perfusion in most series. However, several investigators have demonstrated failure of complete portomesenteric-gastrosplenic disconnection at this stage: this is a technical failure of the surgeon. The coronary, epiploic, umbilical, omental, and colonic collaterals should all be deliberately interrupted. Any significant portaprival collaterals present in the first month after operation time will progressively enlarge, to the detriment of perfusion. In addition, it has been shown there is a 20% incidence of nonoccluding thrombus within the portal vein in the early postoperative phase and a 4% incidence of total thrombosis. The natural history of nonoccluding thrombus is resolution over the next few months, but the cost is more rapid development of collaterals and, in 10%, progression to total thrombosis.[75]

Later follow-up angiography shows a more confusing picture. The controversy revolves around whether or not portal perfusion is maintained. Nabseth et al.,[38] Vang et al.,[55] Maillard et al.,[43] and Belghiti et al.[76] have shown progressive formation of collaterals, reduction of portal vein diameter, and decreasing prograde portal flow after DSRS. Their data, however, do not show total loss of all portal perfusion: 62% still exhibit some, although diminished, hepatopetal portal flow. On the other side of the controversy, the Emory University group has shown continuing portal perfusion of some degree in 69% of a group of 13 patients a mean of 7.5 years after operation.[46] There is no question that collaterals will develop from the high-pressure portal to the low-pressure splenic system over time. The time course and the effect of this development on portal perfusion and liver function are currently being studied.

A recent study has helped to clarify this controversy.[29] Twenty-four patients with cirrhosis were evaluated angiographically prior to and serially for 1 year after DSRS. Seven of the eight nonalcoholic patients retained the same portal perfusion at 1 year, with only one patient losing perfusion. On the other hand, 12 of the 16 patients with alcoholic cirrhosis lost portal perfusion over the same time interval. Thus, the disease etiology appears to play a major role in whether or not portal perfusion is retained. The mechanism of this significant difference awaits explanation. Analysis of the cause of cirrhosis in the studies cited above shows that "loss of perfusion" is seen predominantly in alcoholic cirrhotics, while the studies showing "continuing perfusion" have a higher proportion of nonalcoholic patients. This observation raises more questions than it answers, but nevertheless opens an investigative pathway to study pathophysiology.

The final comment on angiographic studies following DSRS relates to the development of portal-splenic collateral pathways. Unpublished data obtained by our group show that virtually all patients develop some collaterals and that these follow distinct patterns. The three main routes are transpancreatic, left gastric/short gastric, and the transverse mesocolon. The origin of these collaterals is off the superior mesenteric/portal vein junction over a 4–6-cm distance, often from the right side of the vessel. The final common pathways to these three routes are into the splenic vein (1) where it is still connected to the pancreas, (2) to the superior ramus through short gastric veins, and (3) to the inferior ramus of the splenic vein.

The transpancreatic pathway (see Fig 1) acts as a siphon, draining all pancreatic venous blood to the shunt. While such collaterals do not completely decompress the portal hypertension—portal venous perfusion is maintained in 60%—they do deprive the liver of pancreatic hormones. This may be an important factor in the significant reduction in liver volume seen after DSRS. Splenopancreatic disconnection, described above, is currently being evaluated as a means of preventing this siphon.

NONANGIOGRAPHIC ASSESSMENT OF PORTAL PERFUSION AFTER DSRS.—Mathie and associates[77] assessed hepatic tissue perfusion intraoperatively before and after DSRS by the krypton washout technique. They showed a mean perfusion of 116 ml/minute/100 gm of liver before DSRS and 108 ml/minute/100 gm of liver after DSRS. In contrast, the single patient they studied with portal vein clamping showed a reduction from 161 to 40 ml/minute/100 gm of liver during portal vein occlusion.

Reichle and Owen[42] evaluated seven patients prior to and early after DSRS by lipoidal droplet velocity in the portal vein. The mean preoperative portal flow, 929 ± 147 ml/minute, was not significantly reduced at 899 ± 271 ml/minute following DSRS. Their data on mesocaval shunts, however, showed a drop in hepatofugal flow from a preoperative mean of plus 772 ± 177 ml/minute to minus 1,021 ± 310 ml/minute after operation.

Both of these short-term studies document and quantify continuing portal perfusion immediately after DSRS. The advent of increasingly sensitive, and presumably accurate, ultrasound/Doppler techniques may offer a practical method for the measurement of portal venous blood flow in longitudinal studies.[78]

LIVER BLOOD FLOW.—Guharay et al.[79, 80] measured total liver blood flow before and after DSRS in two groups of patients using BSP. In the 10 patients with portal vein thrombosis there was no significant change in total liver blood flow. In three adult patients with cirrhosis and three with noncirrhotic portal fibrosis they documented a mean preoperative flow of 1,178 ± 291 ml/minute which did not fall significantly after DSRS (1,131 ± 243 ml/minute).

Reichle and Owen,[42] using continuous infusion (ICG) in six patients, measured mean total liver blood flow at 1,501 ± 347 ml/minute prior to DSRS, with no significant fall at 1,310 ± 337 ml/minute after operation. In contrast, the data of Maillard et al.,[43] who also used ICG, showed a significant reduction from 1,250 ± 475 ml/minute prior to shunt to 790 ± 240 ml/minute 2–5 weeks after DSRS. This fall was more marked in patients with the higher preoperative flows. The use of ICG, with decreasing extraction by the liver in the context of advancing disease, coupled to the vagaries of hepatic vein sampling, may in part account for these discrepancies.

A new approach to the measurement of nutrient liver blood flow using low-dose galactose clearance[81] has been applied to shunt patients and illustrates the complexity of their hemodynamic changes.[29] Evaluation of 24 patients with cirrhosis prior to and 1 year after DSRS showed distinctly different hemodynamic patterns between the 16 alcoholic and 8 nonalcoholic patients. Portal perfusion, judged angiographically, was retained by 88% of the nonalcoholic but by only 25% of the alcoholic patients at 1 year. What were the other hemodynamic differences? The cardiac output was not significantly different between groups prior to DSRS (mean ± SD, 6.9 ± 1.7 L/minute): 1 year after operation the nonalcoholic group showed no change (7.3 ± 2.8 L/minute), but there was a significant ($P < .05$) increase in cardiac output in the alcoholic group (10.0 ± 3.5 L/minute). In parallel with this finding, the nonalcoholic group showed no change in liver blood flow (1,045 ± 269 → 964 ± 169 ml/minute), but the alcoholic cirrhotic patients showed a mild ($P < .07$) increase in flow (1,133 ± 265 → 1,339 ± 406 ml/minute) at 1 year. When flow is looked at in combination with the galactose elimination capacity (GEC), an index quantifying the flow required to perform specific function can be expressed as flow per unit of GEC (ml/mg GEC). Application of this index to the above data shows that nonalcoholics maintain a virtually normal flow/function relationship at 1 year (3.0 ± 0.7 → 3.1 ± 0.5 ml/mg GEC); on the other hand, the alcoholics require significantly ($P < .05$) more flow to perform the same function at 1 year (3.5 ± 0.9 → 4.6 ± 1.5 ml/mg GEC). A possible interpretation of this difference is that loss of portal perfusion, and therefore reliance purely on hepatic arterial flow, necessitates a greater total liver blood flow to maintain hepatocyte integrity. This study highlights several points: (1) the hemodynamics of cirrhotic patients are exceedingly complex and are altered by DSRS, (2) disease etiology plays some role in the hemodynamic response in cirrhosis, and (3) the quality of liver blood flow, i.e., portal versus hepatic arterial, is probably more important than the quantity.

The full picture on changes in liver blood flow after DSRS is not yet complete. It must be considered in light of the changes induced by cirrhosis itself and must be evaluated with full knowledge and awareness of disease etiology, hepatocyte function, and systemic hemodynamic changes.

Hepatic Function

The aim of DSRS is to preserve the functional hepatocyte mass at the preoperative level. For an operation with such a specific functional goal, there is a dearth of quantitative data to support that goal. In this section we summarize the available data on how far quantitative hepatic function alters after DSRS, based largely on our own experience.

Routine liver test results (bilirubin, albumin, prothrombin time, SGOT, alkaline phosphatase) were analyzed before DSRS and at hospital discharge in 300 patients in our series.[33] The bilirubin level rose significantly, from 1.4 to 3.3 mg/dl ($P <$ .001), and the prothrombin time rose from 1.6 to 1.9 seconds greater than control ($P <$ .02). There was no significant change in albumin or the liver enzyme levels. Similar findings have been reported by others.[54] Regression analysis of the preoperative variables to determine which variables, singly or combined, correlate with survival showed that albumin correlated best ($P <$ .006), followed by the prothrombin time ($P <$ .007) and Child's class ($P <$ .02). However, these variables are indicators of liver damage rather than of liver function, and assessment of continuing liver function must include quantitative data defined by specific rate processes occurring in the liver.

NITROGEN METABOLISM.—The liver is centrally involved in the metabolism of protein. The main factors that will alter protein metabolism in chronic liver disease are liver blood flow, transport from blood into hepatocyte, intact metabolic pathways, and total hepatic mass. Each of these factors is disturbed in cirrhosis, the degree of disturbance depending on the stage of the disease, the degree of fibrosis, and loss of portal perfusion. Protein is initially broken down into its constituent amino acids, which are then degraded by individual pathways, nitrogen being removed from the carbon skeletons early in the process. Half of this nitrogen is metabolized through ammonia prior to its entry into the final common path of urea synthesis in the Krebs-Henseleit cycle; the other half is transaminated and enters the urea cycle as aspartic acid. Quantitative assessment of nitrogen metabolism can therefore be determined either from the individual amino acids, in a fasting state or in response to a stimulus, ammonia metabolism, or from rates of urea synthesis.

AMINO ACIDS.—Progressive cirrhosis is characterized by an abnormal fasting amino acid profile, with elevation of the aromatic amino acids (AAA) phenylalanine, tyrosine, and tryptophan and depletion of the branched chain amino acids (BCAA) valine, leucine, and isoleucine. Reduction of the BCAA/AAA ratio has been etiologically linked to encephalopathy by some,[82] while others relate this to the severity of hepatocellular damage.[83] Data from Fischer et al.[72] have shown that early after DSRS, the BCAA/AAA fell from 1.97 to 1.60. This change is not statistically significant and is brought about entirely by a rise in phenylalanine and tyrosine levels. Our own data[46] obtained from randomized patients 7 years after operation show the BCAA/AAA ratio in 12 patients with DSRS to be 1.8, while in seven patients with total shunts it was 1.3. This difference was primarily due to higher AAA levels in the total shunt patients.

The ability to metabolize individual amino acids can be quantified following a standard protein load.[84] Measurement of plasma amino acids serially for 6 hours after a 40-gm protein meal will give amino acid data in the same manner as a glucose tolerance test. Use of this method has shown that in cirrhosis, there is a parallel decline in the ability to utilize aromatic and branched chain amino acids.[84] Data are not yet available on the changes in individual amino acid metabolism serially after DSRS.

AMMONIA.—Elevated fasting plasma levels of ammonia have long been considered an index of impaired nitrogen metabolism in liver disease. Technical difficulties in sample collection, handling, and assay have combined to raise doubts as to its validity.[85] Ammonia data must be interpreted in light of diet, medications, and catharsis; each can be manipulated to alter plasma ammonia levels. Measurements under standardized conditions, such as for the protein load studies above, probably provide a clinically useful index of protein metabolism. Maintenance of portal venous hypertension in the intestinal bed is an important factor in reducing ammonia absorption. Evaluation of the changes in fasting ammonia and D-xylose absorption after selective and nonselective shunts showed no changes in

DSRS patients but a significantly greater D-xylose absorption and higher ammonia in the total shunt patients.[86] The ammonia changes significantly correlated with the increased D-xylose uptake, leading to the conclusion that altered intestinal absorption may be an important factor in alterations in cerebral function after shunt surgery.

UREA SYNTHESIS.—This metabolic process occurs exclusively in the liver, so its measurement is a true liver function test.[87] Kinetic tracer methodology allows direct measurement of de novo urea synthesis by infusion of ^{14}C urea.[88] Concomitant infusion of amino acids to stimulate urea production enables one to quantify the significant impairment in this process that occurs in cirrhosis.

Measurement of urea synthesis before and early after DSRS showed no significant decrease in the rate of synthesis.[67] This contrasts to the significant reduction ($P < .05$) in the concomitantly studied group of total shunt patients. The same patients studied a mean of 3 years after DSRS showed a small but not significant further reduction of this index.[28]

GALACTOSE ELIMINATION CAPACITY.—Functional hepatocyte mass can be measured by GEC. The maximal removal rate of galactose from plasma can be calculated after giving 30 gm intravenously, saturating the metabolic pathway, and measuring the plasma concentration of galactose from 20 to 60 minutes. The normal GEC is 450–550 mg/minute.[23]

This index is not significantly changed by DSRS when evaluated at 1 year.[29] Evaluation of 24 patients with cirrhosis showed a mean ± SD GEC of 345 ± 99 mg/minute prior to shunt and of 316 ± 78 mg/minute 1 year after shunt. In contrast to the hemodynamic studies presented earlier, there was no significant difference in GEC between alcoholic (337 ± 99 → 305 ± 69 mg/minute) and nonalcoholic patients (362 ± 98 → 324 ± 93 mg/minute). However, as previously noted, the alcoholic patients, who as a group had significant reduction in portal perfusion, had a significantly higher flow per unit GEC at 1 year than the nonalcoholics ($P < .05$). GEC measurement 7 years after shunt in our patients prospectively randomized to receive either DSRS or total shunt showed better retained hepatocyte function in the 12 DSRS patients (324 ± 87 mg/minute) than in the seven patients with a patent total shunt (253 ± 63 mg/minute).[46]

The hepatic function data now available to quantitatively assess the effect of shunt surgery shows that DSRS preserves hepatocyte function better than a total portal-systemic shunt. However, all such data must be understood in the context of chronic liver disease, which is often progressive, and data interpretation must take into account the natural history of that process.

Conclusion

The available data lead us to the following conclusions on the current state of selective variceal decompression:

1. Selective variceal decompression is best achieved by DSRS but can be achieved by other means.

2. It prevents recurrent gastroesophageal variceal bleeding.

3. Survival is significantly improved in patients with nonalcoholic cirrhosis and schistosomiasis compared to total shunt procedures in the same populations.

4. Survival in alcoholic cirrhotics is not significantly improved compared to survival after total shunt procedures in the same population.

5. The incidence of encephalopathy is significantly lower than after total shunt procedures, regardless of disease etiology.

6. Portal venous perfusion is retained in 60% of patients at 1 year and in some patients for up to 12 years.

7. Hepatic function is better preserved after DSRS than after total shunts.

8. Portomesenteric to gastrosplenic collaterals develop after selective shunts. New surgical methods may minimize this complication.

Acknowledgment

Work was supported in part by NIH grant No. 5–R01–AM15736.

REFERENCES

1. Warren W.D., Zeppa R., Foman J.J.: Selective transplenic decompression of gastroesophageal varices by distal splenorenal shunt. *Ann. Surg.* 166:437–455, 1967.

2. Resnick R.H., Iber F.L., Ishihara A.M., et al.: A controlled study of the therapeutic portacaval shunt. *Gastroenterology* 67:843–857, 1974.

3. Jackson F.C., Perrin E.B., Felix R.W., et al.: A clinical investigation of the portacaval shunt: V. Survival analysis of the therapeutic operation. *Ann. Surg.* 174:672–701, 1974.

4. Rueff B., Prandi D., Degos F., et al.: A controlled study of the therapeutic portacaval shunt in alcoholic cirrhosis. *Lancet* 1:655–659, 1976.

5. Hassab M.A.: Gastroesophageal decompression and splenectomy in the treatment of esophageal varices in bilharzial cirrhosis: Further studies with a report on 355 operations. *Surgery* 61:169–176, 1967.
6. Johnson G., Dart C.H., Peters R.M., et al.: Hemodynamic changes with cirrhosis of the liver: Control of arteriovenous shunts during operation for esophageal varices. *Ann. Surg.* 163:692–701, 1966.
7. Warren W.D., Muller W.H.: A clarification of some hemodynamic changes in cirrhosis and their surgical significance. *Ann. Surg.* 150:413–420, 1959.
8. Warren W.D., Restrepo J.E., Respess J.C., et al.: The importance of hemodynamic studies in management of portal hypertension. *Ann. Surg.* 158:387–394, 1963.
9. Mikkelsen W.P., Edmondson H.A., Peters R.L., et al.: Extra- and intra-hepatic portal hypertension without cirrhosis (hepatoportal sclerosis). *Ann. Surg.* 162:602–608, 1965.
10. Conn H.O., Lindenmuth W.W.: Prophylactic portacaval anastamosis in cirrhotic patients with esophageal varices: Interim results, with suggestions for subsequent investigations. *N. Engl. J. Med.* 279:725–732, 1968.
11. Jackson F.C., Perrin E.B., Smith A.G., et al.: A clinical investigation of the portacaval shunt: II. Survival analysis of the prophylactic operation. *Am. J. Surg.* 115:22–42, 1968.
12. Resnick R.H., Chalmers T.C., Ishihara A.M., et al.: The Boston Interhospital Liver Group: A controlled study of the prophylactic portacaval shunt. A final report. *Ann. Inter. Med.* 70:675–688, 1969.
13. Reynolds T.B., Donovan A.J., Mikkelsen W.P., et al.: Results of a 12-year randomized trial of portacaval shunt in patients with alcoholic liver disease and bleeding varices. *Gastroenterology* 80:1005–1011, 1981.
14. Drapanas T., LoCicero J., Dowling J.B.: Hemodynamics of the interposition mesocaval shunt. *Ann. Surg.* 181:523–533, 1975.
15. Fulenwider J.T., Nordlinger B.M., Millikan W.J., et al.: Portal pseudoperfusion, an angiographic illusion. *Ann. Surg.* 189:257–268, 1979.
16. Stipa S., Ziparo V., Anza M., et al.: A randomized controlled trial of mesentericocaval shunt with autologous jugular vein. *Surg. Gynecol. Obstet.* 153:353–356, 1981.
17. Linton R.R., Ellis D.S., Geary J.E.: Critical comparative analysis of early and late results of splenorenal and direct portacaval shunts performed in 169 patients with portal cirrhosis. *Ann. Surg.* 154:446–459, 1961.
18. Johnson W.C., Widrich W.C., Ansell J.E., et al.: Control of bleeding varices by vasopressin: A prospective randomized study. *Ann. Surg.* 183:369–376, 1977.
19. Clark A.W., Macdougall B.R.D., Westaby D., et al.: Prospective controlled trial of injection sclerotherapy in patients with cirrhosis and recent variceal hemorrhage. *Lancet* 2:552–554, 1980.
20. Paquet K.J., Fleig W.E.: Sclerotherapy of esophageal varices, in Papp J.P. (ed.): *Endoscopic Control of Gastrointestinal Hemorrhage.* Boca Raton, Fla., CRC Press, 1981.
21. Galambos J.T.: Cirrhosis: *Major Problems in Internal Medicine.* Philadelphia, W.B. Saunders Co., 1979.

22. Nordlinger B.M., Nordlinger D.F., Fulenwider J.T., et al.: Angiography in portal hypertension: Clinical significance in surgery. *Am. J. Surg.* 139:132–141, 1980.
23. Henderson J.M., Millikan W.J., Wright L., et al.: Quantitative estimation of metabolic and hemodynamic hepatic function: The effects of shunt surgery. *Surg. Gastroenterol.* 1:77–85, 1982.
24. Warren W.D., Millikan W.J.: Selective transsplenic decompression procedure: Changes in technique after 300 cases. *Contemp. Surg.* 18:11–32, 1981.
25. Henderson J.M., El Kishen M.A., Millikan W.J., et al.: Stenosis of distal splenorenal shunt: Management by balloon dilatation. *Surg. Gynecol. Obstet.* 157:43–48, 1983.
26. Warren W.D.: Control of variceal bleeding. Reassessment of rationale. *Am. J. Surg.* 145:8–16, 1983.
27. Warren W.D., Millikan W.J., Henderson J.M., et al.: Selective variceal decompression after splenectomy or splenic vein thrombosis: With a note on splenopancreatic disconnection. *Ann. Surg.,* to be published.
28. Rikkers L.F., Rudman D., Galambos J.T., et al.: A randomized, controlled trial of the distal splenorenal shunt. *Ann. Surg.* 188:271–282, 1978.
29. Henderson J.M., Millikan W.J., Wright-Bacon L., et al.: Hemodynamic differences between alcoholic and nonalcoholic cirrhotics following distal splenorenal shunt: Effect on survival? *Ann. Surg.* 198:325–334, 1983.
30. Starzl T.E., Porter K.A., Francavilla J.A., et al.: A hundred years of the hepatotrophic controversy: Hepatotrophic factors. *Ciba Found. Symp.,* pp. 111–138, 1978.
31. Hoshino S., Inoue H., Igooi T., Honda K.: Experience with left gastric venacaval shunt for esophageal varices. *Jpn. J. Surg.* 131:130–134, 1983.
32. Henderson J.M., Warren W.D.: Current status of the distal splenorenal shunt. *Semin. Liver Dis.* 3:251–263, 1983.
33. Warren W.D., Millikan W.J., Henderson J.M., et al.: Ten years portal hypertensive surgery at Emory: Results and new perspectives. *Ann. Surg.* 195:530–542, 1982.
34. Zeppa R., Hensley G.T., Levy J.V., et al.: The comparative survival of alcoholics versus nonalcoholics after distal splenorenal shunt. *Ann. Surg.* 187:510–514, 1978.
35. Brittan R.C.: The clinical effectiveness of selective portal shunts. *Am. J. Surg.* 13:506–511, 1977.
36. Martin E.W., Molnar J., Cooperman M., et al.: Observations of fifty distal splenorenal shunts. *Surgery* 84:379–383, 1978.
37. Langer B., Patel S.C., Stone R.M., et al.: Selection of operation in patients with bleeding esophageal varices. *Can. Med. Assoc. J.* 118:369–372, 1978.
38. Nabseth D.C., Johnson W.C., Widrich W.C., et al.: Splenorenal shunts in portal hypertension. *J. Cardiovasc. Surg.* 20:201–207, 1979.
39. Busutill R.W., Brin B., Tompkins R.K.: Matched control study of distal splenorenal and portacaval shunts in the treatment of bleeding esophageal varices. *Am. J. Surg.* 138:62–67, 1979.
40. Soper N.J., Rikkers L.F.: Effects of operations for variceal hemorrhage on hypersplenism. *Am. J. Surg.* 144:700–703, 1982.

41. Reiner D.S., Kaminski D.L.: Comparative evaluation of selective and nonselective peripheral portosystemic shunts for treatment of variceal hemorrhage. *Am. J. Surg.* 144:704–710, 1982.
42. Reichle F.A., Owen O.E.: Hemodynamic patterns in human hepatic cirrhosis: A prospective randomized study of the hemodynamic sequelae of distal splenorenal (Warren) and mesocaval shunts. *Ann. Surg.* 137:13–21, 1979.
43. Maillard J.N., Flamant Y.M., Hay J.M., et al.: Selectivity of the distal splenorenal shunt. *Surgery* 86:663–671, 1979.
44. Widrich W.C., Robbins A.H., Johnson W.C., et al.: Long-term followup of distal splenorenal shunts: Evaluation by arteriography, shuntography, transhepatic portal venography and cinefluorography. *Radiology* 134:341–345, 1980.
45. Zeppa R.: Discussion of hemodynamics after DSRS. *Ann. Surg.* 198:332, 1983.
46. Henderson J.M., Millikan W.J., Wright L., et al.: Distal splenorenal shunt or interposition H-graft: Results of a prospective randomized study at 7 years, abstracted. *Gastroenterology* 82:1230, 1982.
47. Warren W.D.: Reflections on the early development of portacaval shunts. *Ann. Surg.* 191:519–527, 1980.
48. Voorhees A.B., Chaitman E., Schneider S., et al.: Portalsystemic encephalopathy in the noncirrhotic patient: Effect of portal systemic shunting. *Arch. Surg.* 107:659, 1973.
49. Warren W.D., Millikan W.J., Smith R.B., et al.: Noncirrhotic portal vein thrombosis: Physiology before and after shunts. *Ann. Surg.* 192:341–349, 1980.
50. Rodgers B.M., Talbert J.L.: Distal splenorenal shunt for portal decompression in childhood. *J. Pediatr. Surg.* 14:33–37, 1979.
51. Maksoud J.G., Mies S.: Distal splenorenal shunt (DSS) in children: Analysis of the first 21 consecutive cases. *Ann. Surg.* 195:401–405, 1982.
52. Kallio H., Lempiren M.: Distal shunt for portal hypertension. *Ann. Chir. Gynaecol.* 70:1–4, 1981.
53. Kieninger G.: Der distal splenorenale Shunt. *Chirurg* 52:717–721, 1981.
54. Marni A., Trojsi C., Belli L.: Distal splenorenal shunt: Hemodynamic advantage over total shunt and influence on clinical status, hepatic function and hypersplenism. *Am. J. Surg.* 142:281–284, 1981.
55. Vang J., Simert G., Hansson J.A., et al.: Results of a modified distal splenorenal shunt for portal hypersplensim. *Ann. Surg.* 185:224–228, 1977.
56. Mosimann R., Loup R.: Efficacy and risks of the distal splenorenal shunt in the treatment of esophageal varices. *Am. J. Surg.* 133:163–198, 1977.
57. Cuschieri A.: Selective decompression for bleeding esophageal varices in patients with preparenchymal blocks. *J. R. Coll. Surg. Edinb.* 26:229–231, 1981.
58. Funovics J.M., Fritsch A., Appel W.H., et al.: Ergebnisse mit den distalen-splenorenalen Shunt nach Warren. *Langenbecks Arch. Chir.* 354:81–88, 1981.
59. Maillard J.N., Flamant Y., Hay J.M.: Operation de Warren et anastomose spleno-renale distale sans deconnexion. *Chirurgie* 108:523–525, 1982.

60. Fekete F., Belghiti J., Gremier P., et al.: L'anastomose de Warren: Resultats cliniques et angiographiques. *Acta Chir. Lug.* 30:5–16, 1983.
61. Saubier E.C., Partansky C., Gouillat C.: Early postoperative angiographic control of the Warren procedure in 40 patients. *World J. Surg.* 6:765–770, 1982.
62. Marqios C., Gertsch P., Mosimann R.: Control angiographique, endoscopic et manometrique a long terme des anastomoses spleno-renales distales don Warren. *Helv. Chir. Acta* 49:633–636, 1982.
63. Prete F., Neri V., Montemurro S., et al.: L'anastomosi spleno-renale distale nel trattamento dell'ipertensione portale. *Minerva Chir.* 37:405–408, 1982.
64. Raia S.: *Descompressao Portal Selectiva: Na Esquistossomose Mansonica.* Universidade de Sao Paulo, Brazil, 1978.
65. Habashi A.H.F.: Transsplenic decompression of oesophageal varices by selective distal splenorenal shunt. *J. Egypt. Med. Assoc.* 60:23–28, 1977.
66. Machado A.L., Filho J.E.B., Campos A.B., et al.: Selective distal splenorenal shunts: Technique and results. *Am. J. Surg.* 142:281–284, 1981.
67. Galambos J.T., Warren W.D., Rudman D., et al.: Selective and total shunts in the treatment of bleeding varices: A randomized controlled trial. *N. Engl. J. Med.* 295:1089–1095, 1976.
68. Reichle F.A., Fahmy W.F., Golsorkhi M.: Prospective comparative clinical trial with distal splenorenal and mesocaval shunts. *Am. J. Surg.* 137:13–21, 1979.
69. Langer B., Rotstein L.E., Stone R.M., et al.: A prospective randomized trial of the selective distal splenorenal shunt. *Surg. Gynecol. Obstet.* 150:45–48, 1980.
70. Villamil F., Redeker A., Reynolds T., et al.: A controlled trial of distal splenorenal and portacaval shunts, abstracted. *Hepatology* 1:557, 1981.
71. Conn H.O., Resnick R.H., Grace N.D., et al.: Distal splenorenal shunt vs portal-systemic shunt: Current status of a controlled trial. *Hepatology* 1:151–160, 1981.
72. Fischer J.E., Bower R.H., Atamian S., et al.: Comparison of distal and proximal splenorenal shunts: A randomized prospective trial. *Ann. Surg.* 194:531–544, 1981.
73. Smith R.B., Warren W.D., Salam A.A., et al.: Dacron interposition shunts for portal hypertension: An analysis of morbidity correlates. *Ann. Surg.* 192:9–17, 1980.
74. Ottinger L.W.: The Linton splenorenal shunt in the management of the bleeding complications of portal hypertension. *Ann. Surg.* 196:664–668, 1982.
75. Henderson J.M., Millikan W.J., Chipponi J., et al.: The incidence and natural history of thrombus in the portal vein following distal splenorenal shunt. *Ann. Surg.* 196:1–7, 1982.
76. Belghiti J., Grenier P., Nouel O., et al.: Long-term loss of Warren's shunt selectivity: Angiographic demonstration. *Arch. Surg.* 116:1121–1124, 1981.
77. Mathie R.T., Toouli J., Smith A., et al.: Hepatic tissue perfusion studies during distal splenorenal shunt. *Am. J. Surg.* 140:384–386, 1980.
78. Saito M., Ohnishi K., Nakayama T., et al.: Ultrasonic measurements of

portal and splenic vein blood flows and their velocities in normal subjects and patients with chronic liver disease, abstracted. *Hepatology* 3:812, 1983.

79. Guharay B.N., Sain P., Ramerjee D., et al.: Direct splenocaval shunt for selective docompression of portal hypertension in children. *Surgery* 87:271–279, 1980.

80. Guharay B.N., Sain P., Sengupta K.P., et al.: Graft interposition splenocaval shunt for total or selective decompression of portal hypertension. *Surgery* 83:164–170, 1978.

81. Henderson J.M., Kutner M.H., Bain R.P.: First-order clearance of plasma galactose: The effect of liver disease. *Gastroenterology* 83:1090–1096, 1982.

82. Fischer J.E., Rosen H., Ebeid D., et al.: The effect of normalization of plasma amino acids on hepatic encephalopathy in man. *Surgery* 80:77–91, 1976.

83. Morgan M.Y., Marshall A.W., Milson J.P., et al.: Plasma amino acid patterns in liver disease. *Gut* 23:362–370, 1982.

84. Ibrahim S., Millikan W.J., Henderson J.M., et al.: Branched-chain amino acid tolerance following oral protein load in normal and cirrhotic subjects. *Surg. Forum* 34:36–38, 1983.

85. Ansley J.D., Isaacs J.W., Rikkers L.F., et al.: Quantitative tests of nitrogen metabolism in cirrhosis: Relation to other manifestations of liver disease. *Gastroenterology* 75:570–579, 1978.

86. Rikkers L.F.: Portal hemodynamics, intestinal absorption, and post shunt encephalopathy. *Surgery* 94:126–133, 1983.

87. Rudman D., Difulco T.H., Galambos J.T., et al.: Maximal rates of excretion and synthesis of urea in normal and cirrhotic subjects. *J. Clin. Invest.* 52:2241–2249, 1973.

88. Rypins E.B., Henderson J.M., Fulenwider J.T., et al.: A tracer method of measuring rate of urea synthesis in normal and cirrhotic subjects. *Gastroenterology* 78:1419–1424, 1980.

Horizons in Surgical Oncology

JOHN M. DALY, M.D., F.A.C.S.* AND JEROME J.
DECOSSE, M.D., F.A.C.S.†

*Associate Attending Surgeon, and †Chairman, Department of Surgery,
Memorial Sloan-Kettering Cancer Center; and *Associate Professor of
Surgery, and †Professor and Vice-Chairman, Department of Surgery,
Cornell University Medical College, New York, New York*

Introduction

In the review that follows, it is important to recognize that
the domain of surgical oncology extends far beyond the confines
of the operating room and the application of manipulative techniques. The surgical oncologist is interested in all aspects of
the patient with neoplasia: the causes and precursors of cancer,
multimodal treatment of the cancer patient, evaluation of the
systemic consequences of neoplasia, and provision for maximum rehabilitation of the patient to normal life. The operating
room is the site of much progress such as advances in technical
concepts, remodeling of older operations, perfusion and infusion
techniques, and multimodal treatments such as intraoperative
radiation therapy. Advances in surgical oncology derive from
advances in surgery in general. Here the cardiorespiratory care
of the very sick patient, the control of infection, and important
advances in repletion and nutrition have been prominently led
by surgeons.

Surgical oncologists have maintained a major interest in tumor immunology, perhaps from their strengths in transplanta-
tion biology. They have sustained a loyalty to the discipline of
surgical pathology, perhaps from its inseparable linkage with
understanding the natural history of cancer. Surgical oncolo-

117

0065-3411/84/0018-0117-0144-$04.00

gists have increasing awareness and understanding of interactions of operative intervention with chemotherapy and radiation therapy. The field is moving toward more multidisciplinary care and it behooves the surgical oncologist to understand basic concepts of radiation therapy and chemotherapy.

Surgeons see patients with early cancer and its precursors. Therefore, surgeons have the opportunity to address risk for development of cancer. Surgeons are led into epidemiology and into secondary prevention, therefore these areas may also be regarded as elements of surgical oncology.

PREVENTION

Most common cancers have identifiable precursors. These precursors and their respective cancer include: leukoplakia and squamous cancer of the oral cavity; squamous metaplasia and cancers in the lung or esophagus; atrophic gastritis and cancer of the stomach; adenomas and large bowel cancer; cervical dysplasia and cervical cancer; endometrial hyperplasia and endometrial cancer; keratoses and basal and squamous skin cancer; and, dysplastic nevi and malignant melanoma. A cause-and-effect relationship between the presence of the precursors and direct degeneration into neoplasia is arguable, but circumstantial evidence for more than simple association is strong. For example, Morson and other pathologists involved with large bowel neoplasia conclude that most and perhaps all large bowel cancers are preceded by large bowel adenomas.[1]

One of the horizons of surgical oncology is addressed to the earlier and more accurate identification of these precancerous tumors and earlier eradication of them. There is evidence that aggressive removal of large bowel adenomas decreases the incidence of large bowel cancer. The presence of these lesions also provides a setting for efforts at pharmacologic control, an area of increasing interest called chemoprevention.

Whether or not the precursor lesion evolves directly to cancer, the presence of these precursors is a biomarker of high risk. The presence of these precursor lesions and the identification of genetic risk defines a subpopulation of persons who merit more intensive surveillance. Here screening studies are moving from mass population studies toward concentration of these resources on those patients with identifiable risk factors.

Patients with these risk factors lead the surgical oncologist still further into the background of human neoplasia to address epidemiology and carcinogenesis. The subject is complex and cannot be addressed at length. Numerous surgeons have contributed at the Surgical Forum to our understanding of carcinogenesis and to other immunologic and biochemical aspects of neoplasia. Many surgeons have contributed to the epidemiology of cancer. Perhaps the foremost surgical contributor of this century was Alton Oshsner who early on recognized the association between cigarette smoking and carcinoma of the lung.

Diagnostic Modalities

The advent of computerized tomography and ultrasound have added to our armamentarium in the diagnosis of neoplastic disease. Nuclear magnetic resonance is on the horizon. Advances in imaging have allowed preoperative observations to be made that were not previously possible. Computerized tomographic scans, particularly critical in neuro-oncology, are also used widely for screening for tumors at other sites. With respect to abdominal tumors, ultrasound, which avoids radiation exposure, may have equal or greater utility than CT scanning.

The advent of these imaging techniques has led to the development of invasive radiology, an increasing dynamic field. Invasive radiology has resulted in major advances in transcutaneous biopsies, the management of intra-abdominal and intrahepatic abscess and in the development of drainage techniques such as percutaneous nephrostomy. The application of these techniques will surely be extended during coming years.

Mammography remains a major tool in the diagnosis of breast cancer. Here the development of techniques that provide less radiation exposure has led to extension of recommendations regarding annual mammography for all women older than age 40 years. It can be expected that the introduction of even safer techniques will further extend the recommendations for mammography.

Another important area of technologic evolution in surgical oncology is in flexible endoscopy. The techniques of flexible upper and lower gastrointestinal endoscopy are well known. Choledochoscopy is being applied more widely. With the development of these diagnostic techniques, conversion to therapeutic utility has also become increasingly widespread. The operation, colotomy and polypectomy, has all but disappeared as endoscopists have developed greater skills in the removal of adenomas in the large bowel. Laparoscopy has provided increasing usefulness in the diagnosis of intra-abdominal disease, thus lessening the need for exploratory laparotomy. The application of laser technology through the endoscope for control of gastrointestinal bleeding is an area of active interest.

Surgical Staging

The earliest role of the surgeon in the multidisciplinary management of the patient with cancer is to establish a tissue diagnosis. Depending on the clinical diagnosis and tumor size, incisional or excisional biopsy has provided the classic approach. To be assured of the most representative tissue in the diagnosis of lymphoma, the largest lymph nodes compatible with good surgical judgment are removed with intact capsules in order to allow definite pathologic diagnosis of cell type, which influences prognosis. In selecting a site for lymph node biopsy, preference should be given to the cervical and supraclavicular areas, with the axillary area as a second choice. The specimen should be submitted in an unfixed state to the pathologist; antigenic cell surface markers have become increasingly important in the diagnosis of lymphoma. More recently, core-needle biopsy and fine-needle aspiration biopsy have been used to establish a histologic diagnosis for solid tumors. The latter approach has shown remarkable accuracy for thyroid and breast cancer. When guided by ultrasound, pancreatic malignancy can be confirmed by fine-needle aspiration biopsy with little morbidity. Lymph node scintiscans are being developed that will more accurately help to define the extent of disease and aid in treatment planning.

STAGING LAPAROTOMY

Since 1967, staging laparotomy and splenectomy have been evaluated for its indications and usefulness in patients with Hodgkin's and non-Hodgkin's lymphoma; controversy still exists regarding its true role in the management of these patients. Undoubtedly, staging laparotomy with splenectomy is a valuable tool to define precisely intra-abdominal sites of disease in patients with Hodgkin's disease. However, the decision to use laparotomy in staging should be closely linked to the therapeutic approach used in managing the patient and his disease; this is the focal point of the controversy regarding the indications for staging laparotomy. One must bear in mind that if modalities such as chemotherapy continue to improve without an accompanying increase in complications or if other effective systemic types of therapy develop, the need for complete, accurate staging by laparotomy will diminish.

Among 139 patients with Hodgkin's disease reviewed by Gamble et al., the radiologists' interpretation of a normal lymphangiogram was confirmed by staging laparotomy in 134 instances.[2] In only five patients was histologic evidence of Hodgkin's disease found in lymph nodes that had been interpreted as normal. However, Hodgkin's disease was found outside of the visualized lymphatic system in 40 of these 139 patients. Management of these patients was then based on findings from staging laparotomy.

Sutcliffe et al. performed staging laparotomy in 68 patients with untreated stage I and stage II supradiaphragmatic presentation.[3] Twenty-four (36%) patients had their clinical stage changed; 20 patients were downstaged because occult disease was found in the abdomen. In four patients, a preoperative assessment of intra-abdominal disease was incorrect, and the clinical stage was upgraded. Thirty-three percent of clinical stage I patients and 34 percent of clinical stage II patients were changed to pathologic stage III. These authors noted that accurate preoperative assessment of splenic involvement was difficult; only 70% of clinically enlarged spleens were involved pathologically, whereas normal-sized spleens contained Hodgkin's disease in 40% of cases. Sutcliffe et al. concluded that the use of total nodal and splenic irradiation would negate any value of staging laparotomy. It would also result in overtreating many patients appearing with localized disease and would represent undertreatment in the 10% of patients who have stage IV disease established by staging laparotomy.

If total nodal irradiation is the planned mode of treatment for stage I and stage II disease without evidence for abdominal involvement, then staging laparotomy and splenectomy has only limited value, such as in identifying liver involvement. In such a case, percutaneous liver biopsy is a much simpler method to document hepatic invasion from Hodgkin's disease. DeVita et al. and Beretta et al. have used peritoneoscopy to stage patients with Hodgkin's disease more completely; they found liver involvement in 16% and 6% of their patients, respectively.[4, 5] This procedure was a safe and economical way to establish stage IV disease with liver involvement mainly in patients with extensive nodal involvement shown by lymphangiogram.

Thus, although the specific indications for staging laparotomy and splenectomy in patients with Hodgkin's disease are controversial, it is generally agreed that staging laparotomy and splenectomy provides the most accurate documentation of the presence or absence of intra-abdominal disease. Staging laparotomy with splenectomy is useful when it serves as a guide to treatment decision. Future advances in surgical staging may involve greater use of peritoneoscopy, invasive radiology, and development of radioisotope-labeled monoclonal antibodies for scintiscan determination of extent of disease.

Nutritional Abnormalities in the Cancer Patient

The consequences of malnutrition in the cancer patient are severe. Warren, in a classic article published in 1932, reviewed a large series of autopsies and found that cancer cachexia alone accounted for at least 22% of all cancer deaths.[6] Protein-calorie deprivation not only leads to obvious weight loss, but also to compromise of less obvious visceral and somatic protein vital to enzymatic, structural and mechanical function. Impairment of immunocompetence and increased susceptibility to infection may result. Poor wound healing, wound dehiscence, prolonged intestinal ileus, extended hospitalization, and increased mortality may result from surgical procedures in the malnourished patient. Proper doses of chemotherapy or radiotherapy may be withheld because the threshold of toxicity is reduced in malnourished cancer patients.

Changes of body composition accompany weight loss in cancer patients. Cohn has used prompt gamma neutron activation to evaluate total body nitrogen and the whole body counter to determine total body potassium in cancer patients.[7] In cancer patients who lost weight, total body potassium was diminished out of proportion to total body nitrogen; the loss of potassium in these patients was primarily from the skeletal muscle component of body cell mass (only 45% of total body nitrogen is in muscle as opposed to 80% of total body potassium). There were significant losses of total body fat, but even with such severe wasting, retention of a large proportion of body fat was evident. Further studies of body composition of cancer patients using these direct methods are presently under way.

The signs and symptoms of malnutrition have prognostic significance. Costa determined that weight loss was a better predictor of death in lung cancer patients than performance status, tumor histology, or type of chemotherapy used.[8] DeWys found that median survival in patients with significant weight loss was less than in those without it.[9] Within categories of performance status, weight loss was associated with decreased median survival, particularly in favorable categories of performance status. A multivariant prognostic nutritional index has been described that identifies surgical patients at risk for operative complications and death based on the level of depression of nutritional determinants such as serum albumin level, serum transferrin level, triceps skinfold thickness, and delayed cutaneous hypersensitivity.

NUTRITIONAL SUPPORT

Before 1973, the use of nutritional support in cancer patients was deterred by two major considerations; possible alterations of tumor growth and the potential for infectious complications. Copeland and Dudrick found no discernible tumor stimulation in 406 cancer patients supported with total parenteral nutrition (TPN).[10] Most of these patients, however, received antineoplastic therapy during the course of their nutritional support. Mullen et al. found no increase in tumor protein synthesis in a group of patients with tumors of the upper gastrointestinal tract who received preoperative nutritional support.[11] Schwartz also noted that tumors generally grow at the maximal rate and that the addition of hyperalimentation had no effect.[12] Thus, the weight of evidence at present is that exogenous nutrients have little selective effect on tumor growth in human beings.

A second complicating factor from TPN in cancer patients involves the use of indwelling catheters in patients who may be immunosuppressed. Copeland et al. demonstrated that catheter-related sepsis occurred in only 2.3% of cancer patients receiving TPN.[10] Patients with head and neck cancer had the highest rates of catheter-related sepsis due to draining oral, pharyngeal, and tracheotomy secretions on the catheter insertion site. Although there may be an increased rate of subclavian vein thrombosis in selected cancer patients, there is no evidence at present that the complication rate from this procedure is different in cancer patients than in other patients.

RESULTS OF NUTRITIONAL SUPPORT

Improved tumor response and decreased host toxicity from the use of TPN during administration of chemotherapy has been shown in animal studies. Reynolds and Daly found that there was greater tumor inhibition in malnourished rats who received methotrexate after two days of nutritional repletion compared to protein-depleted rats.[13] With the infusion of added nutrient substrates, it is possible that dormant tumor cells in malnourished animals are induced to replicate in synchrony with other tumor cells and are thus more susceptible to cycle-specific drugs. In animals, both the pharmacokinetics of chemotherapeutic drugs, as well as host toxicity to these agents, are modulated by the host's nutritional status. Souchon noted less gastrointestinal toxicity from chemotherapy and increased survival in parenterally fed versus orally fed animals.[14] Applying a committed granulocyte-macrophage progenitor cell assay, Gamelli found significant decreases in the progenitor cell population of the bone marrow in protein-starved mice and an increase in toxicity to a single dose of 5-FU after a single day of repletion in similar starved mice.[15] The same dose of 5-Fluorouracil (5-FU) was given to protein-starved animals that were repleted for four days. Here an increased kill of progenitor cells could not be demonstrated, suggesting that both the length and timing of nutritional repletion was important.

Results in animal studies and retrospective clinical reports regarding the use of TPN with chemotherapy have not been reproduced in prospective randomized clinical studies. Samuels studied the role of TPN during chemotherapy for stage III testicular cancer.[16] The TPN-treated group experienced less weight loss, but gastrointestinal side effects from the therapy were not decreased. Popp studied a group of patients with advanced diffuse lymphoma with and without TPN during their chemotherapy.[17] No difference in tolerance of any specific drug was observed between the two groups. Lanzotti noted no advantage to giving TPN with chemotherapy in terms of increasing patient survival or tumor response rate in patients with non-oat cell lung cancer.[18]

Results of prospective randomized trials have been encouraging in patients undergoing surgery for gastrointestinal tract neoplasms. Mueller noted a statistically significant reduction in major postoperative complications and mortality for patients with gastrointestinal cancer who received ten days of preoperative nutritional support compared with control patients (Table 1).[19] Heatley gave preoperative TPN for 7 to 10 days to patients with stomach or esophageal cancer and found a decrease in postoperative wound infections in the TPN-treated group.[20]

The ability of a patient to respond to nutritional therapy as an adjunct may depend more on his ability to respond to antineoplastic treatment. For nutritional support to show a real difference in small populations of patients, a dramatic increase in survival would need to be demonstrated. In cancer with a dismal prognosis, this may be difficult to do. If the primary oncologic treatment is ineffective, benefit from adjuvant nutritional support may be obscured. Although definitive answers on improvements in tumor response or patient survival is awaited, it is clear from these clinical studies that malnutrition should not preclude appropriate surgery or delivery of adequate amounts of chemotherapy or radiotherapy. In addition, no cancer patient who is undergoing antineoplastic therapy should be

TABLE 1.—PREOPERATIVE TOTAL PARENTERAL NUTRITION IN PATIENTS WITH GI CANCER: PROSPECTIVE RANDOMIZED TRIAL

	CONTROLS	TPN (10 DAYS PREOP)
Number of patients	59	66
Change in mean body weight (kg) (from admission to operation)	−1	+2
Number of patients with postoperative complications	19(32%)	11(16%)
Postoperative mortality	11(19%)	3(4%)*

*Difference between TPN group and controls is significant ($P < .005$).
From Muller et al.: *Lancet,* 1:68, 1982

allowed to become severely malnourished during treatment. Future directions of nutritional support in cancer patients will relate to studies of biochemical epidemiology related to carcinogenesis and its prevention or inhibition. Nutritional support of the patient with an established tumor will focus on methods of longer-term enteral nutrition with substrates that may selectively starve the tumor while maintaining host nutritional status.

Decision for Operation

A decision for curative operation presupposes that the tumor is localized or confined regionally, the area of the tumor can be encompassed by regional excision, distant metastases cannot be documented, and that the tumor is appropriately treated by operation.

Given a decision for a curative operation, the extent of the surgical procedure must then be defined. In principle, an *en bloc* resection should be performed, encompassing the primary tumor, the regional lymph nodes, and the intervening lymphatic channels. Perhaps this principle is best illustrated by operations for large bowel cancer where the regional lymphatics of the colon (but not the rectum) course in one direction with major arteries and veins. This principle is less applicable in the rectum where lateral spread and the limiting confines of the lateral pelvic wall preclude a wide margin. Similarly, the principle is less applicable for breast cancer where multiple pathways of lymphatic spread are well recognized.

As a result of these concepts and partly due to emergence of earlier-stage disease, the extent of various operations for cancer are undergoing change. This "remodeling" is, perhaps, best illustrated in breast cancer where the trend is toward a modified radical mastectomy or local excision with adjuvant radiation therapy and adjuvant chemotherapy. The therapeutic value of regional node dissection in breast cancer has been questioned by some; performed properly, node dissection at least establishes the data base for precise staging for other adjuvant treatments.

Operative intervention is used for palliative treatment in a variety of settings. Bypasses are performed around obstructed viscera, for example, gastrojejunostomy may be necessary for obstructing carcinoma of the stomach, choledoduodenostomy or choledochojejunostomy for a carcinoma of the pancreas obstructing the common bile duct, or nephrostomy may be necessary to vent an obstructed ureter. Plastic Celestin tubes may be inserted through an obstructing esophageal carcinoma, and colon diversion may be performed for obstructing large bowel cancer.

The use of cytoreductive surgery, or reduction of tumor burden, is controversial. This concept may be most relevant in ovarian cancer where deliberate removal of as much ovarian tumor as possible may enhance the patient's response to subsequent chemotherapy or radiation therapy. Cytoreductive operations also may be valid in the treatment of some childhood tumors, such as neuroblastoma or Wilm's tumor.

The extent of an operation should be dictated by precise staging. In many instances, a regional node dissection is carried out to remove all lymph nodes in anticipation of metastases in some. With precise staging, and with the presence of effective chemotherapy, operative intervention may be more selective. For example, the traditional management of nonseminoma germ cell tumor of the testis has been radical orchiectomy and radical retroperitoneal lymph node dissection extending to the renal vasculature. The predictability of a normal beta subunit of human chorionic gonadotrophin (β HCG) and a normal alpha fetoprotein (αFP) with normal CT scans and ultrasound, backed by effective chemotherapy should dissemination occur, may now permit only radical orchiectomy without node dissection in those patients who are normal by these determinants. More precise pretreatment planning for patients with tumors traditionally treated by an initial operation is a main objective of current research.

Organ Sites

BREAST

If no evidence of distant metastasis is found, the treatment plan for the patient with breast cancer is determined, often in consultation with a radiation therapist and a medical oncologist, by the anatomical location of the lesion, its physical characteristics, and evidence of regional metastases. In the past, excision of the suspicious lesion and frozen section examination was performed under general anesthesia immediately before mastectomy. More recently, needle biopsy or needle aspiration for cytology is performed under local anesthesia for tumors 1.5 cm or larger to establish the diagnosis of cancer; discussion is then undertaken with an informed patient regarding the proposed method of therapy.

Baker reported 153 consecutive biopsies performed under local anesthesia.[21] Patients found to have breast cancer were admitted to the hospital within 1 to 3 days for definitive treatment. An increase in local recurrence was not observed compared with patients who had an open breast biopsy immediately before mastectomy. In patients with stage I and stage II tumor, modified radical mastectomy continues to be the treatment of choice. Laterally located cancer with metastases to the axillary lymph nodes may be associated with internal mammary or supraclavicular lymph node metastases in as many as 25% to 30% of cases; consequently, radiation therapy is often used to treat these areas (called peripheral lymphatic radiation therapy). Medially located cancer is associated with internal mammary lymph node metastases in 30% of patients; if axillary metastases are also present, the incidence of internal mammary metastases rise to about 50%. At some centers, internal mammary nodes are biopsied before selecting radiation therapy as an adjuvant treatment.

Other approaches have been used to treat patients with small (< 2 cm) cancers of the breast. Veronesi et al. compared radical mastectomy with quadrantectomy, axillary dissection, and radiotherapy in 701 patients with breast cancers measuring less than 2 cm in diameter (Table 2).[22] Local chest wall or ipsilateral recurrence of tumor and actuarial survival of the patients were similar in both groups. The longest patient follow-up, however, was 7.5 years with a mean follow-up of 3 years.

In the NASBP trials, Fisher et al. found no difference in treatment failures between the group treated with total mastectomy plus local-regional radiation and the radical mastectomy group.[23] Calle et al., however, reported on 120 patients with breast tumors less than 3 cm in diameter and without adenopathy who underwent "lumpectomy" and radiotherapy.[24] The rate of local-regional recurrence was 13% at five years and

TABLE 2.—BREAST CARCINOMA < 2 cm: RANDOMIZED
TRIAL OF RADICAL MASTECTOMY VS. QUADRANTECTOMY,
AXILLARY DISSECTION, AND RADIOTHERAPY*

	MASTECTOMY	QUADRANTECTOMY, AXILLARY DISSECTION, AND RADIOTHERAPY
Number of patients	349	352
Primary diameter 1 cm (%)	44.4	46.0
Mean age (yr)	50.9	50.1
Local recurrences	3	1
Secondary primary tumors		
Ipsilateral breast	0	4
Contralateral breast	5	9
Distant metastases	30	22

*Median follow-up = 3 years
Adapted from Veronesi V., et al.: *N. Engl. J. Med.* 305:6–11, 1981.

20% at ten years, with 14 of 16 cases requiring secondary surgery. This latter study emphasizes the importance of adequate follow-up to assess local recurrence of breast cancer.

Sixty percent of cases of recurrent breast cancer occur within two years after mastectomy. If the initial local treatment for breast cancer is proper, local chest wall recurrence rates should be less than 5% in stage I disease and less than 10% in stage II disease. Breast reconstruction should probably not be performed simultaneously with mastectomy in women with invasive breast cancer and should be discouraged for at least two years postoperatively in women who have had axillary lymph node metastases. The major criticism of immediate breast reconstruction is the potential for delay in diagnosing local chest wall recurrence. The best defined role for immediate breast reconstruction may be in the treatment of in situ breast cancer. The cancer surgeon should plan his ablative operative procedure with reconstruction in mind. A transverse incision, preservation of the nerves to the pectoralis major and a subcuticular closure are helpful steps. The surgeon should not, however, compromise the chance for local control of disease in order to preserve cosmetic appearance.

ESOPHAGUS AND STOMACH

Operative therapy for carcinoma of the esophagus has been associated with mortality rates as high as 30%. The high mortality can be attributed to patient factors such as preexisting cardiopulmonary disorders and malnutrition and to anatomical factors such as the lack of an esophageal serosal covering, location of the tumor, and extent of spread. Ellis and Gibb described 82 patients with esophageal cancer who underwent resection with a mortality of 3% and a complication rate of 15%.[25] They emphasized the importance of esophagogastric reconstruction and perioperative hyperalimentation to reduce complications in these debilitated patients. Daly et al. reviewed the results of surgical therapy for esophageal cancer at M.D. Anderson Hospital from 1960 to 1980 and noted a significant decrease in perioperative complications after 1973; the reduced complication rate was associated with aggressive preoperative nutritional support.[26] This reduction in surgical morbidity was especially apparent in those patients who were supported preoperatively and postoperatively with TPN.

In addition to intensive preoperative support to reduce postoperative complications, adjunctive radiotherapy and/or chemotherapy have been applied in an attempt to reduce local recurrence and increase patient survival. Increased survival has been noted in patients treated with surgical resection plus perioperative radiation therapy compared with controls who had had surgery only. Marks et al. reported that preoperative radiation treatment to 4,500 rad produced tumor sterilization in 3% and reduction to in situ carcinoma in 10% of 101 patients.[27] Kelson et al. treated 53 patients with preoperative combination chemotherapy consisting of cis-platinum (3 mg/kg), bleomycin (10 units/sq m IV loading dose and 10 units/sq m 24 hours × 4-day infusion), and vindesine (3 mg/sq m) for one to two chemotherapy cycles and noted a partial response in 29 patients (55%).[28] In addition, the surgical resectability rate was increased to 82% compared with 54% in controls who had had only preoperative radiation treatment.

LIVER

Advances in anesthesia, blood replacement, and surgical technique have made major hepatic resection feasible with a low morbidity and a mortality of less than 3%. Patients with primary hepatoma and solitary metastatic cancer, of which carcinoma of the large bowel is the most common primary source, should be evaluated for possible curative resection. Adson and Van Heerden reported a 20% to 30% survival after resection of even large hepatic metastases.[29] If liver function tests indicate any degree of hepatocellular malfunction, the patient is a borderline candidate for a major resection. Other contraindications such as advanced age or other organ system disease may mitigate against resection.

Isotopic hepatic scanning combined with serum alkaline phosphatase and CEA are the most effective tests for screening patients for liver disease. Arteriography outlines the arterial blood supply to the liver and may define deposits of metastatic cancer. Variations in origin in the right and left hepatic artery must be known preoperatively, particularly if hepatic artery ligation or infusion chemotherapy is contemplated as an alternate procedure to resection. Computerized axial tomography and ultrasonography are sensitive tests to identify small metastatic deposits, and are much better in detecting tumor in the lateral segment of the left hepatic lobe than is arteriography.

Disappointment with results of systemic chemotherapy for treatment of colorectal hepatic metastases has led to renewed interest in regional infusion chemotherapy of the liver. This method of treatment is particularly applicable in this disease since isolated metastases to the liver occur in 30% of patients. In 1959, Sullivan et al. introduced the method of chemotherapy by continuous hepatic arterial infusion and noted "significant objective tumor regression" in 13 of 16 patients.[30] Clinical benefit was described in ten of these patients.

Unfortunately, use of external catheters placed either at operation or by the Seldinger technique has resulted in high complication rates including catheter displacement, sepsis, and gastrointestinal hemorrhage.[31] Reed et al. reported a 76% tumor response rate in 88 patients with metastatic large bowel cancer with a median response duration of 12 months.[32] However, complications in this series were frequent with an operative mortality of 12% and catheter-related morbidity of 24%. Using the Seldinger technique of external catheter placement, Oberfield et al. reported complications in 48 of 60 patients (80%).[33] Complete or partial hepatic artery thrombosis occurred in 39% and catheter displacement in 33% of patients. Reed et al. reported 109 patients who had external hepatic artery catheters placed by either the Seldinger technique or direct insertion at laparotomy. Complications resulting in interruption in therapy occurred in 35% of patients: catheter clotting, arterial thrombosis and catheter displacement accounted for the majority of complications.

The liver has a dual blood supply from the hepatic artery and portal vein. Transportation of micrometastases to the liver occurs through the portal venous system. Anatomical studies, however, have suggested that the hepatic artery is the predominant blood supply for hepatic macrometastases from the large bowel. These results have been suggested both by human autopsies with dye injection studies and by animal-tumor models. Documentation in vivo in patients, however, has been limited by available techniques to measurement of vascularity of metastatic colorectal tumors in the liver. From a technical standpoint, it is easier to place a catheter into the portal venous system than the arterial system. In addition, a significant reduction in complications of chemotherapy, such as gastritis and gastroduodenal ulceration, has been suggested when infusion chemotherapy was provided via the portal venous route. Storer and Akin, for example, reported no hepatic toxicity following prolonged infusion with relatively large doses of 5-FU through the portal vein.[34] Several investigators have combined ligation of the hepatic artery with infusion of the portal vein to augment tumor response; they have noted an improvement in patient survival.

In 1980, Buchwald et al. reported the use of an implantable infusion pump for regional hepatic arterial chemotherapy in five patients.[35] Several investigators have found a tumor reponse rate ranging from 29% to 83% with minimal catheter-related complications using this implantable infusion device. An implantable pump delivery system offers several potential advantages: (1) reduction in catheter-related sepsis; (2) ease of drug administration; and (3) greater patient acceptance without bulky external devices. Direct placement negates the problem of catheter displacement and allows better determination of the presence or absence of intra-abdominal extrahepatic disease; the presence of disease should exclude pump placement.

In studies at our institution, 60 consecutive adult patients with hepatic metastases from large bowel cancer underwent operative placement of implantable pumps and surgical staging of liver involvement. Extrahepatic tumor was either absent or was resected (Table 3). Nine patients underwent pump placement and simultaneous colon resection. Postoperatively, patients received FUDR, 0.3 mg/kg per day for 2 weeks alternating with heparinized saline for 2 weeks. Tumor response occurred in 48% of patients with a median survival not reached but beyond 17 months in patients with less than 60% hepatic involvement. Operative complications were minimal with patients being discharged an average of 8 days after operation having started their chemotherapy. Chemotherapeutic complications were predominantly gastrointestinal with gastritis or ulceration found in 45% of patients. Patient survival was inversely related to the extent of hepatic tumor involvement as assessed intraoperatively.

Recently, studies have suggested that prediction of patient survival can be based on a variety of preoperative determinants related to degree of tumor involvement in the liver. Determinants such as serum albumin, alkaline phosphatase, LDH levels and patient performance status have been used to predict length of patient survival. However, the ability to predict tumor response to chemotherapy treatment is limited. The degree of tumor vascularity on hepatic arteriogram was suggested to be predictive of the tumor's response to arterial infusion chemotherapy. Hepatic metastases from large bowel cancer have a consistent hypovascular pattern on hepatic angiograms, which limits the ability of this test to predict tumor response to treatment.

Technetium-99 macroaggregated albumin scans of hepatic arterial flow have been suggested to predict tumor response in patients with hepatic metastases from large bowel cancer treated by arterial infusion chemotherapy.

We evaluated the utility of preoperative arteriograms and

TABLE 3.—INFUSION CHEMOTHERAPY TREATMENT RESULTS (n = 60)

	PREVIOUSLY UNTREATED	FAILED PREVIOUS TREATMENT
N	38	22
Mean Age (yrs)	61	60
Median % liver disease	40	45
Median Preop CEA (ng/ml)	64	36
Tumor Response (evaluable pts.)	19/32 (60%)*	6/21 (29%)

*$P < .02$

immediate postoperative arterial flow scans with Technetium-99 macroaggregated albumin to predict tumor response in patients who underwent operative placement of hepatic pumps for chronic infusion chemotherapy. In 46 evaluable patients, arteriograms had a sensitivity of 56% and a specificity of 46% in predicting tumor response to treatment. In 39 patients with increased tumor uptake of Technetium-99 macroaggregated albumin, this finding predicted tumor response with a sensitivity of 92% and a specificity of 77%. A rim sign of decreased central tumor uptake with increased uptake around the tumor, which was present in eight patients, was found to be of no value in predicting response to chemotherapy. Thus, prediction of tumor response to either regional or systemic infusion treatment may depend on host-tumor biologic and vascular determinants that may be applied in patient selection for infusional treatment.

Although operative and technical complications with the use of a surgically placed catheter and implantable pump have been minimal, complications of chemotherapy have been substantial. The major chemotherapy-related morbidity has been gastrointestinal with gastritis and duodenitis in 10% to 60% of patients and gastroduodenal ulceration in 6% to 11% of patients. Narset et al. described gastric ulceration in eight patients during intrahepatic arterial infusion with 5-FU.[36] Ensminger et al. found gastritis in 60% and ulcers in 8% among 60 patients receiving chronic hepatic arterial chemotherapy.[37] It is unclear how often endoscopy was applied in their series of patients and an underestimate of the problem is possible. Chemical hepatitis with elevated bilirubin levels has been reported in 15% to 33% of patients receiving regional hepatic infusion chemotherapy; however this complication is associated with little morbidity.

Large Bowel

Preoperative preparation of the patient with colorectal carcinoma requires thorough assessment by physical examination, radiographic methods, and endoscopic techniques to determine the size, mobility, and histology of the primary tumor. Synchronous cancers of the large bowel have been noted in approximately 4% of patients. Currently, there is little debate regarding the need for antibiotic prophylaxis in addition to a vigorous mechanical preparation, but controversy remains as to antibiotic choice, the length of time for perioperative administration, and whether antibiotics should be given orally or intravenously.

Good surgical judgment is necessary when operating on any part of the large bowel, but is required most when dealing with carcinoma of the rectum and rectosigmoid. The surgical oncologist should provide the best opportunity for cure and local control of disease combined with the least chance of postoperative morbidity, mortality, and loss of function. Sphincter-saving procedures should not be performed if the chance for local control is jeopardized. Malignant tumors within 5–6 cm of the anal verge, which invade through the muscularis propria, should almost always be removed by abdominoperineal resection. Cancer above this level can often be managed with a low anterior resection, transsacral excision or a colo-anal procedure. Use of automated suturing devices may allow a lower anastomosis to be performed but there is no evidence that safety is improved. It should be emphasized that attempts to perform a low anastomosis should not compromise a wide pelvic dissection.

Morson et al. have demonstrated the applicability of *local* excision for *early* cancer of the rectum in lesions that undergo complete excision with low-grade histology and with tumor confined to the submucosal plane of the bowel wall without lymphatic or vascular invasion.[38] This approach to small polypoid distal rectal cancer is preferable to electrosurgical diathermy, which destroys histologic markings and makes staging impossible. In our hands, electrocoagulation has been useful only as palliation for selected patients.

Adjunctive radiation therapy may be indicated in some patients since surgical therapy alone yielded the high recurrence rates in Dukes' C lesions with high-grade histology, size greater than 4 cm and distance within 5 cm of the dentate line compared with other rectal tumors. The Veterans Administration Surgical Oncology Group has entered 5,100 patients over a period of 23 years into a series of trials in an effort to improve survival and decrease recurrence.[39] Preoperative radiation therapy (2,000–2,500 rad) reduced the percentage of patients having positive lymph nodes from 44% to 26% in those with a low-lying cancer requiring abdominoperineal resection. A second trial involving the application of 3,150 rad is currently under way. The Gastrointestinal Tumor Study Group has shown a significantly longer disease-free interval in rectal cancer patients given radiation therapy (4,000 rad) and chemotherapy postoperatively, but morbidity was increased by this approach.

Preoperative radiation therapy has been suggested to increase resectability, prevent seeding, and destroy cancer cells outside the operative field. Alternatively, postoperative radiotherapy spares those patients with more favorable pathologic lesions and can be given to a surgically defined area, but complications, particularly small bowel radiation enteritis, may be more frequent.

Approximately two thirds of recurrences from colorectal cancer are detected within 18 months of surgical resection. Therefore, follow-up examination is extremely important if one is to identify recurrent tumor when it can be treated and possibly cured. Minton and Martin studied prospectively 18 patients who underwent second-look procedures based on elevated plasma CEA levels.[40] Thirteen patients had localized disease, four patients had distant metastases, and in one patient no tumor was discovered. Attiyeh and Stearns performed a second-look laparotomy in 32 asymptomatic patients with significant elevation of the CEA: recurrent tumor was documented in 89%; liver metastases were evident in 18 patients of whom seven had curative resections. Local abdominal disease was found in 15 patients with curative resection attempted in nine.[41] Use of repeated physical examination, endoscopic and radiographic examination, and serum markers such as CEA has improved the surgeon's ability to resect locally recurrent disease. Whether cure rates are improved by this "recovery" surgery is being evaluated currently.

ADULT SOFT TISSUE SARCOMA

Soft tissue sarcomas in adults may grow to a large size without detectable metastases. Prognosis has been shown to correlate with tumor size, site, histologic type, and degree of differentiation. Tumors that are small (less than 5 cm), superficial (not extending beyond the superficial fascia), and low grade are grouped together as tumors with a favorable prognosis. Tumors that are large (more than 5 cm), deep (extending beyond the superficial fascia), and high grade have a poor prognosis.

Traditionally, soft tissue sarcomas have been treated surgically. Experience, however, has shown that simple excision results in a local recurrence rate of 90% due to a "pseudocapsule," an outer sheath of viable tumor cells that is stripped away and left behind. Local recurrence rates approximate 39% after wide excision, 25% after muscle group soft part resection and 7% to 18% after radical amputation. In contrast, the local recurrence rate after radical radiation treatment alone was shown to be 66%.

In a series of 82 patients with liposarcoma of the extremity seen from 1949–67 an en bloc resection of the muscle group was applied in some patients and radical amputation in others; the overall rate of local recurrence was 27%.[42] Ten patients had a wide soft part resection and adjunctive radiation therapy; the local recurrence rate was 10%. Lindberg et al. also emphasized use of postoperative radiation therapy in "unfavorable" lesions in an attempt to preserve a functional limb.[43] The overall local recurrence rate was 22% with a functional limb preserved in 84% of patients.

In a prospective randomized trial comparing amputation with wide local excision plus radiotherapy, local recurrence occurred in none of 16 patients treated with amputation and in four of 26 undergoing combined treatment.[44] All local recurrences occurred in the thigh, especially in those with positive surgical margins. Finally, Eilber et al. reported a 3% local recurrence rate for extremity sarcomas treated with intra-arterial doxorubicin, and 3,500 rad of external beam radiotherapy followed by radical en bloc resection of the primary tumor with limb salvage.[45]

Thus, conservative surgery plus adjunctive radiation therapy with or without chemotherapy decreases local recurrence when *complete* operative removal with adequate surgical margins has been accomplished. Ideally, the surgeon and radiation therapist should plan their approach together. In order to minimize local recurrence, all areas of the operative site should be irradiated. Brachytherapy has special appeal since very high doses of radiation can be delivered to a precise field within a short time. Brachytherapy combined with wide regional resection has resulted in only one local recurrence in 23 patients.[46]

The surgical approach to the management of soft tissue sarcomas must take into account the previously described prognostic criteria. Adequate tumor material usually obtained by open surgical biopsy should lead to an accurate histologic diagnosis by permanent section before treatment decisions can be made. Care must be taken to plan the biopsy approach so as not to compromise later surgical extirpative therapy. Ultrasound and CT scan of the extremity are useful in defining the gross limits of the tumor and proximity to vital structures. Angiography may be necessary to define both vascular supply and involvement of major blood vessels by sarcoma.

Vascular Access

Safe, readily available angioaccess in the cancer patient is essential for administration of fluids, chemotherapeutic agents, antibiotics, and a variety of other medications. Patients who receive periodic outpatient chemotherapy may require vascular access only temporarily; perioperative surgical patients may require continuous intravenous therapy for days or weeks. Sepsis remains the most serious, potentially lethal complication associated with intravenous therapy, and its prevention is a primary objective in the management of the cancer patient.

Scalp vein needles, short plastic catheters and central venous catheters are the most common instruments for vascular access in cancer patients. Arteriovenous grafts have also been used for long-term intermittent chemotherapy in cancer patients in whom vascular access is difficult. Finally, completely implantable central venous Silastic catheters with plastic reservoirs have recently been reported to provide safe, long-term vascular access with improved patient acceptability.

Scalp vein needles provide short-term intravenous access with the lowest incidence of peripheral phlebitis because the frequent occurrence of infiltration results in a short duration of use. Short plastic cannulas provide more secure infusion sites but their longer duration in situ results in a higher incidence of phlebitis. Use of in-line filtration and simultaneous administration of heparin (1,000u) and hydrocortisone (10 mg) have been shown to reduce the incidence of phlebitis associated with the use of short plastic cannulas. Central venous catheters are indicated to monitor cardiovascular status, to infuse caustic chemotherapeutic agents continuously, and to administer total parenteral nutrient solutions. Complications associated with their use include technical errors such as pneumothorax, infections, and vascular complications such as venous thrombosis. Physician education has been found to reduce technical complications. Welch et al. noted a significant decrease in venous thrombosis with the use of silicon elastomer catheters compared with polyvinyl and polyethylene catheters.[47] Simultaneous administration of low-dose heparin (1000u) has also been shown to reduce catheter-associated venous thrombosis. Daly et al. reviewed a series of 959 central venous catheters used in cancer patients and noted mechanical complications in 16% of subclavian catheters and in 3% of peripherally-inserted catheters.[48] Catheter-related sepsis occurred in 2.9% and 3.6% of subclavian and peripherally-inserted catheters, respectively.

In thrombocytopenic patients or those patients who require long-term (months) vascular access, Silastic right atrial catheters inserted by direct venous cutdown using local anesthesia have provided excellent vascular access with minimal morbidity. Recently developed "double" Silastic catheters have been used in leukemic patients who require chemotherapy, medications, blood products, and hypertonic nutrient solutions administered concomitantly.

Vascular access surgery in cancer patients is rapidly evolving. Current "state of the art" relies on long-term, Silastic, single or double-lumen, right atrial catheters. Other devices, such as the totally implanted access injection port, are proving useful. Future technical advances with these devices will further resolve the difficult problem of finding safe, long-term vascular access in this population.

Reconstructive

The initial use of myocutaneous flaps dates back to the late 19th century but application of these basic principles, mostly by plastic surgeons, has occurred only in recent years. Development of these flaps has been a major innovation in surgery of the patient with cancer. This renaissance of reconstructive techniques has greatly improved the surgical closure of wounds, provided a means for reconstruction of organs such as the breast and cervical esophagus, and contributed to limb-preserving techniques. This is a rapidly evolving area; a few examples can be provided.

The deltopectoral flap with its pectoral portion based axially on perforators from the internal mammary system in the second to fourth intercostal spaces provides a useful illustration. The deltopectoral flap has been widely applied in reconstruction of the oral cavity.

The sternocleidomastoid flap can be used for intraoral reconstruction, external resurfacing, or esophageal reconstruction. The trapezius flap is widely used for resurfacing after head and neck surgery. The pectoralis major flap is an extremely reliable flap with excellent mobility.[49] It is used for reconstruction of the cranio-orbital cavity after resection and can be applied to a variety of other purposes.

Both the latissimus dorsi and the rectus abdominus flaps have been widely used for reconstruction of the breast or other major defects on the thorax and on the abdominal wall. Lower extremity flaps from the tensor fascialata, gracilus, and gastrocnemius have been widely applied to repair defects on the lower limb and in the lower portion of the abdomen.

In addition to musculocutaneous flaps of one sort or another, a complex array of synthetic prostheses have evolved. These have made subcutaneous mastectomy and either immediate or delayed implants more acceptable to patients at high risk for breast cancer and to patients who have had a mastectomy. These prosthetic materials also have utility in facial reconstruction.

Summary

Future horizons in surgical oncology relate to advances in prevention, diagnosis, and treatment of the patient with cancer. New diagnostic modalities may make complete surgical staging unnecessary. Perioperative support of patients given multimodality treatment will become more critical as the limits of surgical resection are reached and combined treatment with radiation and chemotherapy become more frequent. The current treatment of cancer at several organ sites reflects the evolving approach to treat both local and systemic manifestations of the malignancy. Use of intraoperative radiation therapy with electron-beam and/or brachytherapy has been proved safe and future prospective trials will determine efficacy in local control of disease. Finally, proper reconstruction becomes critical as we attempt to rehabilitate cancer patients toward normal function.

REFERENCES

1. Morson B.C., Day D.W.: Pathology of adenomas and cancer of the large bowel, in Decosse O. (ed.): Large Bowel Cancer, New York, Churchill-Livingston, 1981, pp. 34–45.
2. Gamble J.F., Fuller L.M., Martin R.G., et al.: Influence of staging celiotomy in localized presentations of Hodgkin's disease. *Cancer* 35:817, 1975.
3. Sutcliffe B.J., Wrigley P.F.M., Smyth J.F., et al.: Intensive investigation in management of Hodgkin's disease. *Br. Med. J.* 2:1343, 1976.
4. DeVita V.T., Bagley C.M., Goodell B., et al.: Peritoneoscopy in the staging of Hodgkin's disease. *Cancer Res.* 31:1746, 1971.
5. Beretta G., Spinelli P., Pilke F., et al.: Sequential laparoscopy and laparotomy combined with bone marrow in staging Hodgkin's disease. *Cancer Treat. Rep.* 60:1231, 1976.
6. Warren S.: The immediate cause of death in cancer. *Am. J. Med. Sci.* 184:610, 1932.
7. Cohn S.H., Gartenhaus W., Sowitxky A., et al.: Compartmental body composition of cancer patients by measurement of total body nitrogen, potassium and water. *Metabolism* 30:222, 1981.
8. Costa G., Donaldson S.: The nutritional effects of cancer and its therapy. *Cancer* 2:22, 1980.
9. DeWys W., Begg C., Levin P.J.: Prognostic effect of weight loss prior to chemotherapy in cancer patients. *Am. J. Med.* 69:491, 1978.
10. Copeland E.M., Dudrick S.J.: Nutritional aspects of cancer. *Curr. Prob. Cancer*, Vol. 1, No. 3, 1976.
11. Mullen J.L., Buzby G.P., Gertner M.H., et al.: Protein synthesis dynamics in human gastrointestinal malignancies. *Surgery* 87:331, 1980.
12. Schwartz G.F., Breen H.O., Bendon M.L., et al.: Combined parenteral hyperalimentation and chemotherapy in treatment of disseminated solid tumors. *Am. J. Surg.* 121:169, 1979.
13. Reynolds H.M., Daly J.M., Rowlands B.J., et al.: Effect of nutritional repletion on host and tumor response to chemotherapy. *Cancer* 45:3069, 1980.
14. Souchon E.A., Copeland E.M., Watson P. et al.: Intravenous hyperalimentation as an adjunct to cancer chemotherapy with 5-fluorouracil. *J. Surg. Res.* 30:331, 1981.
15. Gamelli R.L., Foster R.S.: Effect of refeeding on chemotherapeutic myeloid toxicity. *Surg. Forum* 30:450, 1981.
16. Samuels M.L., Selig D.E., Ogden S., et al.: IV hyperalimentation and chemotherapy for stage III testicular cancer: a randomized study. *Cancer Treat. Rep.* 65:615, 1981.
17. Popp M.B., Fischer R.I., Simon R.M., et al.: A prospective randomized study of adjuvant parenteral nutrition in the treatment of diffuse lymphoma: effect on drug tolerance. *Cancer Treat. Rep.*
18. Lanzotti V.C., Copeland E.M., George S.L., et al.: Cancer chemotherapeu-

tic response and intravenous hyperalimentation. *Cancer Treat. Rep.* 59:437, 1975.

19. Mueller J.M., Dienst C., Brenner U., et al.: Preoperative parenteral feeding in patients with gastrointestinal carcinoma. *Lancet* 1:68, 1982.

20. Heatley R.V., Williams R.H.P., Lewis M.H.: Preoperative intravenous feeding a controlled trial. *Post. Med. J.* 55:541, 1979.

21. Baker R.R.: Outpatient breast biopsies. *Ann. Surg.* 185:543, 1977.

22. Veronesi V., Saccozzi R., DelVecchio M., et al.: Comparing radical mastectomy with quadrantectomy, axillary dissection and radiotherapy in patients with small cancers of the breast. *N. Engl. J. Med.* 305:6, 1981.

23. Fisher B., Redmond C., Fisher E., et al.: The contribution of recent NASBP clinical trials of primary breast cancer therapy to an understanding to tumor biology. *Cancer* 46:1009, 1980.

·24. Calle R., Pilleron J.P., Schlienger P., et al.: Conservative management of operable breast cancer. *Cancer* 42:2045, 1978.

25. Ellis F.H., Gibb S.: Esophagagastrectomy for carcinoma. *Ann. Surg.* 190:699, 1979.

26. Daly J.M., Massar E., Giacco G., et al.: Parenteral nutrition in esophageal cancer patients. *Ann. Surg.* 196:203, 1982.

27. Marks R.D., Scruggs H.J., Wallace K.M.: Preoperative radiation therapy for carcinoma of the esophagus. *Cancer* 38:84, 1976.

28. Kelson D.P., Bains M., Hilaris B., et al.: Combination chemotherapy of esophageal carcinoma using Cisplatin, Vindesine and Bleomycin. *Cancer* 49:1174, 1981.

29. Adson M.A., Van Heerdon J.A., Major hepatic resections for metastatic colorectal cancer. *Ann. Surg.* 191:576, 1980.

30. Sullivan R.D., Norcross J.W., Watkins E.: Chemotherapy of metastatic liver cancer by prolonged hepatic-artery infusion. *N. Engl. J. Med.* 270:321, 1964.

31. Patt Y.Z., Mavligit G.M., Ghuang V.P., et al.: Percutaneous hepatic arterial infusion (HAI) of mitomycin C and floxuridine (FUDR): an effective treatment for metastatic colorectal carcinoma in the liver. *Cancer* 46:261, 1980.

32. Reed M.L., Vaitkevicius V.K., Al-Sarraf M., et al.: The practicality of chronic hepatic artery infusion therapy of primary and metastatic hepatic malignancies. Ten-year results of 124 patients in a prospective protocol. *Cancer* 47:402, 1981.

33. Oberfield R.A., McCaffrey J.A., Polio J., et al.: Prolonged and continuous percutaneous intra-arterial hepatic infusion chemotherapy in advanced metastatic liver adenocarcinoma from colorectal primary. *Cancer* 44:414, 1979. ,

34. Storer E.H., Akin T.J.: Chemotherapy of hepatic neoplasm via the umbilical portal vein. *Am. J. Surg.* 111:56, 1966.

35. Buchwald H., Grage T.B., Cassilopoulos P.P., et al.: Intraarterial infusion chemotherapy for hepatic carcinoma using a totally implantable infusion pump. *Cancer* 45:866, 1980.

36. Narset T., Ansfield F., Wirtanen G., et al.: Gastric ulceration in patients receiving intrahepatic infusion of 5-fluorouracil. *Ann. Surg.* 186:734, 1977.

37. Ensminger W., Niederhuber J., Gyves J., et al.: Effective control of liver metastases from colon cancer with an implantable system for hepatic arterial chemotherapy. *ASCO Abstract.* 1982.
38. Morson B.C., Bussey H.J.R., Samoorian S.: Policy of local excision for early cancer of the colorectum. *Gut* 18:1045, 1977.
39. Higgins G.A., Donaldson R.C., Humphrey E.W., et al.: Adjuvant therapy for large bowel cancer. *Surg. Clin. North Amer.* p. 1311, 1981.
40. Minton J.P., Martin E.W.: The use of serial CEA determinations to predict recurrence of colon cancer and when to do a second look operation. *Cancer* 42:1422, 1978.
41. Attiyeh F.F., Stearns M.W.: Second-look laparotomy based on CEA elevations in colorectal cancer. *Cancer* 47:2119, 1981.
42. Shiu M.H., Chu F., Castro E.B., et al.: Results of surgical and radiation therapy in the treatment of liposarcoma arising in an extremity. *Cancer* 123:577, 1975.
43. Lindberg R.D., Martin R.G., Romsdahl M.N., et al.: Conservative surgery and postoperative radiotherapy in 300 adults with soft tissue sarcomas. *Cancer* 47:2391, 1981.
44. Rosenberg S.A., Kent H., Costa J., et al.: Prospective randomized evaluation of the role of limb-sparing surgery, radiation therapy and adjuvant chemoimmunotherapy in the treatment of adult soft-tissue sarcomas. *Surgery,* 84:62, 1978.
45. Eilber F.R., Mirra J.J., Grant T.T., et al.: Is amputation necessary for sarcomas? *Ann. Surg.* 192:431, 1980.
46. Shiu M., Turnbull A., Nori D., et al.: Control of locally advanced extremity soft tissue sarcomas by function-saving resection and brachytherapy. *Cancer* 53:6, 1385, 1984.
47. Welch G.W., McKeel D.W., Jr., Silverstein P., et al.: The role of catheter composition in the development of thrombophlebitis. *Surg. Gynecol. Obstet.* 138:421, 1974.
48. Daly J.M., Lawson M., Speir A., et al.: Angioaccess in cancer patients. *Curr. Prob. Cancer* 5:9, 1981.
49. Ariyan S., Cuono C.B.: Use of pectoralis major myocutaneous flap for reconstruction of large cervical, facial or cranial defects. *Am. J. Surg.* 140:503, 1980.

Current Burn Treatment

CLEON W. GOODWIN, M.D.

*Department of Surgery, Cornell University Medical Center,
New York, New York*

THERMAL INJURY continues to be a major cause of morbidity and mortality in the United States, with over 2 million people burned each year.[1] Although most such injuries can be treated on an outpatient basis, approximately 300 persons per million population require hospitalization. Survival and quality of life depend on severity of injury and sophistication of in-hospital treatment. The major improvements in burn treatment followed recognition of the importance of salt-containing fluids in restoring blood volume in the early postburn period and successful control of fatal burn wound infection by topical antimicrobial agents.[2, 3] This improvement in burn mortality is reflected by an increase in the LA_{50} (the extent of burn, expressed as a percentage of the total body surface, associated with a 50% mortality) from 43.0% in 1949 to 63.1% in 1980.[4-6] As the LA_{50} continues to rise to include truly massive burns, new innovations are less likely to result in the major increments in survival typical of the 1940s–1960s. Nevertheless, in the last decade, major aspects of burn treatment have been fruitfully investigated and promise to improve significantly patient care and outcome. These aspects include definition of optimal resuscitation fluid composition, continued improvements in the control of burn wound infections, and the use of artificial skin substitutes.

0065–3411/84/0018–0145–0176–$04.00

Early Care

ASSESSMENT

Burn injury destroys viable cutaneous elements and elicits pathophysiologic alterations in other organ systems which are related to the extent and depth of burn. The consequences of massive fluid loss and extensive tissue destruction determine not only early care but also the incidence of infection and organ dysfunction and nutritional needs. On initial evaluation an adequate history should be obtained, physical examination performed, and burn severity assessed. Most burned patients are alert following injury and can provide information about the circumstances of the injury. Location and time of injury, preexisting diseases, and chronic medications influence clinical evaluation and subsequent treatment. A general physical examination should detect associated injuries and verify airway adequacy, respiratory exchange, and hemodynamic stability.

Burn severity governs the need for hospitalization and subsequent specialized care. Severity is determined by both extent and depth of the burn. Initially, the extent of injury can be estimated by the rule of 9s, in which various anatomical regions of the adult body represent 9% of the body surface area (BSA) or multiples thereof. In children the head accounts for a higher percentage of BSA and the lower extremities for proportionately less. However, the extent of burn is more accurately estimated by the use of BSA charts which partition the body into much smaller portions and adjust relative BSA for age. Partial thickness burns characteristically are pink to light red in color, wet, painful, and usually heal spontaneously. Full-thickness burns are white or translucent, dry, insensate, and require grafting for wound closure. However, initial estimates of burn depth often are not corroborated by the clinical course of healing in up to 50% of patients.[7]

The major factors influencing initial patient disposition are the severity of the burn injury and the presence of associated medical conditions (Table 1). Considerable expertise is required for the safe transport of burned patients.[8, 9] Of paramount importance is direct contact by the referring physician with the surgeon who will be responsible for continuing the patient's

TABLE 1.—Factors Influencing Disposition of the Burned Patient

MINOR BURN INJURY: Can be treated initially on outpatient basis.
Second-degree burn:
    <15% of BSA in adult.
    <10% of BSA in child.
Third-degree burn:
    <2% of BSA.
MODERATE UNCOMPLICATED BURN INJURY: Usually requires hospitalization (general hospital with experience in burn care or specialized burn treatment facility).
Second-degree burn:
    15%–25% of BSA in adult.
    10%–20% of BSA in child.
Third-degree burn:
    2%–10% of BSA.
MAJOR BURN INJURY: Requires hospitalization in a specialized burn treatment facility.
Second-degree burn:
    >25% of BSA in adult.
    >20% of BSA in child.
Third-degree burn:
    >10% of BSA.
Smaller burns with complicating features:
    Extremes of age: <5 or >60
    Burns of hands, face, feet, perineum.
    Chronic alcoholism or drug addiction.
    Inhalation injury.
    Significant preexisting disease.
    Associated trauma.
    Unreliable home environment for small children.
    Child abuse.

care. Adequate hemodynamic stability, airway, ventilation, and peripheral circulation must be established before transport.

PATIENT PREPARATION

Patients with large burns require secure vascular access for the administration of resuscitation fluids. A large-bore cannula should be inserted percutaneously in a large peripheral vein or a central vein. Cutdowns are avoided because of the high incidence of suppurative thrombophlebitis associated with their use. Stainless steel needles are unreliable since they tend to dislodge as the injured extremity swells. While catheter insertion through unburned skin is preferred, placement through the burn wound does not appear to be associated with a higher incidence of infection, and reliability of vascular access takes precedence over the presence of a burn wound. Preference for central venous catheters in recent years appears to have been accompanied by a falling incidence of suppurative thrombophlebitis.[10] Extension of the central venous catheter into the heart is associated with a high incidence of endocarditis, and the tip should be verified roentgenographically to lie in the vena cava.[11, 12] All intravascular cannulas in burned patients are changed every 48–72 hours to minimize catheter-related infection.

A drainage catheter is placed in the bladder to quantify urinary output, since urine production is the most easily measured and reliable index of adequacy of fluid resuscitation. Tetanus prophylaxis is based on the patient's prior immunization status and should proceed according to the guidelines established by the American College of Surgeons.[13] Prophylactic antibiotics have no place in the in-hospital care of burned patients and are associated with the emergence of organisms resistant to multiple antibiotics. During resuscitation, narcotic analgesics should be administered intravenously (IV) in small doses as the patient's mental status and general condition permit. Morphine is an effective agent and is administered to adults in 3–5-mg increments. Analgesics should not be administered subcutaneously, since they are poorly absorbed when the patient is hypovolemic. Following restoration of intravascular volume, rapid absorption of a previously injected narcotic may cause respiratory depression and profound cardiovascular collapse.

Ileus accompanies most serious burn injury, and all such patients should have tube gastric decompression until bowel function returns, as indicated by passage of flatus and stool. Serial endoscopy has defined the natural history of gastroduodenal mucosal ulceration in burned patients.[14–16] Controlled trials have established that control of gastric pH virtually eliminates the complications of Curling's ulcer (perforation and hemorrhage). Following admission, 30 ml of antacid is administered each hour through the nasogastric tube to maintain the gastric pH above 5. The dosage can be increased if gastric acidity persists below this level. In patients who cannot tolerate antacids, cimetidine at a dosage of 400 mg IV every 4 hours is an acceptable alternative.[18]

INHALATION INJURY

Inhalation injury occurs in nearly one third of patients admitted to large burn centers. Carbon monoxide poisoning undoubtedly affects more burned patients than is generally appreciated; the immediate administration of 100% oxygen by emergency medical personnel on the scene constitutes adequate treatment in most patients and may obscure the intensity of intoxication. Carboxyhemoglobin levels over 40% often lead to refractory cardiac failure and CNS toxicity, and most such patients do not survive the resuscitation phase of burn treatment. With the exception of steam inhalation, direct thermal damage to the respiratory tract is rare. Rather, true inhalation injury is a chemical tracheobronchitis arising from the inhalation of products of incomplete combustion. Burns sustained in a closed space or while the patient was experiencing decreased mentation, such as from drug overdosage or alcoholic intoxication, are often associated with inhalation injury. Such patients usually present with burns of the face, mouth, nasal passage, or oropharnx. Although the presence of inhalation injury adversely influences survival in the thermally injured patients, this effect is significant only in patients with injuries between 30% and 60% of the total BSA.[19] In burns exceeding 60% of body surface, the massive extent of the cutaneous injury itself obscures any added effect of inhalation injury on mortality.

Systematic evaluation of the respiratory tree will detect nearly all cases of clinically significant inhalation injury. Upper airway injury progressing to occlusion and asphyxiation is of primary concern during the first 48 hours following burn injury. The supraglottic structures should be examined with a laryngeal mirror or with a flexible bronchoscope that is advanced only far enough to permit adequate visualization of all involved upper airway structures. If injury is present, as evidenced by erythema, edema, or mucosal blebs, additional manipulation of laryngeal structures may precipitate complete occlusion of the airway. Examination below the cords should be continued after an endotracheal tube has been threaded over the flexible bronchoscope. If upper airway injury is present, the tube can be passed through the vocal cords and bronchoscopy can be continued safely. Flexible fiberoptic bronchoscopy will establish the diagnosis in 80%–85% of patients with inhalation injury.[19, 20] The diagnostic accuracy of inhalation injury can be increased by the use of xenon ventilation-perfusion lung scans.[21] This technique is the only method of documenting acute damage to the pulmonary parenchyma. Following IV injection of 100 μCi of ^{133}Xe, scintigraphic detection of regional inequality or retention of isotope in excess of 90 seconds indicates acute damage. Pulmonary function studies will detect additional patients with inhalation injury, but the complexity of the measurements limits such techniques to research-oriented centers. While pulmonary compliance usually is unaffected by inhalation injury, expiratory flow rate is decreased and pulmonary resistance is increased.[22] The combined use of fiberoptic bronchoscopy, xenon lung scan, and pulmonary function studies allows a 96% diagnostic accuracy in the diagnosis of inhalation injury.[19]

Treatment of inhalation injury is guided by the severity of disease. Carefully managed fluid resuscitation and warmed humidified air or oxygen as guided by blood gas measurements may be sufficient for patients with mild inhalation injury. Impending upper airway obstruction must be treated by endotracheal intubation. Tracheostomy is not indicated since the endotracheal cannula usually can be removed within 72 hours in patients with isolated upper airway injury. Bronchodilators are utilized if bronchospasm develops; aminophylline is infused continuously at doses guided by clinical response and serum concentrations. Severe inhalation injury often precipitates respiratory failure with pulmonary edema and bronchopneumonia, and inadequate respiratory exchange is supported by mechanical ventilation. The prophylactic administration of steroids and aerosolized antibiotics to patients with inhalation injury is without effect on subsequent clinical course and may accentuate small airway obstruction and infection.[23, 24] Prophylactic systemic antibiotics likewise offer no protection and promote the emergence of organisms resistant to multiple antibiotics.[25] Secondary infection with bronchopneumonia is common. Antibiotic treatment is dictated by Gram stain, by culture and sensitivity data, and by surveillance patterns of microbial populations for that critical care unit.

PERIPHERAL CIRCULATION

Following thermal injury, fluid accumulates in damaged tissue, and edema soon becomes clinically apparent. Edema formation is accelerated by the large fluid volumes required for adequate resuscitation. Skin with full-thickness destruction will not expand as fluid accumulates beneath the unyielding eschar. If an extremity is encircled by a full-thickness burn, increasing edema formation progressively elevates tissue pressure until blood flow ceases. Ischemia and loss of that limb may occur if adequate circulation is not restored. Distal cyanosis, delayed capillary refill, deep pain, and neurologic deficits suggest vascular compromise but are relatively nonspecific signs in a severely burned extremity. Swelling and coolness of unburned skin distal to the burn are common but are not indications for surgical intervention.[26] Use of the Doppler ultrasonic flow probe greatly increases the accuracy of perfusion assessment, reducing the need for escharotomy by as much as 50%.[27] The posterior tibial pulses in the lower extremities and the palmar arch pulses in the upper extremities should be assessed hourly. Disappearance of the Doppler signal or a progressive reduction of its intensity indicates vascular compromise and the need for decompression. Isotopic scanning of injured extremities may be a useful adjunct to ultrasonic evaluation of blood flow. The washout of intramuscularly injected ^{133}Xe and the accumulation of IV administered technetium 99m pyrophosphate produce characteristic scintigraphic scans in the presence of compromised circulation and have been utilized to guide surgical intervention.[28, 29]

Burned extremities should be elevated immediately following injury and actively exercised for 5 minutes each hour. Such conservative measures will maintain adequate peripheral circulation in many patients with circumferential full-thickness extremity burns. If such measures fail, escharotomy is indicated. The eschar of involved extremities is incised along the midmedial and midlateral lines down to and just through the subdermal fascial attachments. Inadvertent extension into the subcutaneous tissue results in copious bleeding and is avoided. This procedure is carried out at the bedside and requires no anesthesia since eschar is insensate. Pulses may not be restored in patients with deep thermal burns or additional trauma below the level of the investing fascia. Fasciotomy is indicated in these patients, and should be carried out in the operating room after the patient is hemodynamically stabilized. Thoracic escharotomy may be necessary in a rare patient whose chest wall activity is restricted by an encircling deep third-degree burn.

Resuscitation

PHYSIOLOGY OF RESUSCITATION

Heat of sufficient intensity and duration causes coagulation necrosis and cell death. This injury is accompanied by a striking increase in capillary permeability and accumulation of fluid in damaged tissues. Increased vascular leak and edema occur in unburned tissue in patients with burns exceeding 25% of BSA, but the magnitude of these changes is much less than in injured tissues.[30] The hypoproteinemia consequent to burn injury appears to be responsible for the water content changes in unburned tissue.[31] Blalock initially pointed out the intravascular origin of wound edema fluid.[32] With loss of vascular integrity in burned tissues, isotonic fluid shifts from the intravascular compartment into the interstitial space. Plasma proteins, principally albumin, also are lost into the injured tissues, albeit at a slower rate. The composition of edema fluid closely resembles that of plasma with respect to sodium and potassium.[33] Red blood cell (RBC) deficits of 10%–40% commonly occur following burn injury and are caused by direct thermal destruction, wound stasis, and hemorrhage.[34]

As intravascular volume is lost into the burn wound, plasma volume is reduced and cardiac output falls. Loss of plasma volume occurs in excess of RBC deficits, and the hematocrit may rise to 60%–70% of packed cell volume. Although blood pressure remains near normal early after burn injury, further contraction of plasma volume and hemoconcentration soon eventuate in marked hypotension and compromised organ perfusion. In an animal model of a 40% full-thickness burn injury, cardiac output was reduced 35%.[35] Blood flow to the brain, heart, spleen, pancreas, stomach, duodenum, and colon was preserved during the first hours after injury, while flow to the liver, kidney, and small intestine fell 66%, 50%, and 40% below control values. With resuscitation, renal blood flow was restored only after restoration of normal flow to the other major organs. Thus, if renal blood flow is adequate, perfusion to other major organs is likely sufficient, and urinary output remains the most readily accessible index with which to monitor resuscitation.

The restoration of hemodynamic stability by vigorous resuscitation is not accompanied temporally by a return of cardiac output to normal levels. Cardiac output slowly begins to rise with fluid replacement but does not return to preinjury values until 18–24 hours following injury. At the same time, plasma and blood volumes continue to fall for another 12–24 hours and only return to normal levels by 48–54 hours following burn.[36] By this time, cardiac output has increased to supranormal levels, reflecting the onset of postburn hypermetabolism.

The sustained reduction in cardiac output in spite of apparently adequate resuscitation has been ascribed to the presence of a burn-related myocardial depressant factor.[37–39] This possibility was evaluated in a series of young patients with a mean burn size of 57% of BSA and without any associated injuries.[40] Using M-mode echocardiography, indices of cardiac output, left ventricular blood volume, and myocardial contractility were measured serially during the first 48 postburn hours (Table 2). The cardiac index fell by 12 hours after injury and returned to normal by the end of the second postburn day. The depression in cardiac index was parallelled by similar reductions in left ventricular diastolic volume index; as cardiac output rose, so did ventricular blood volume. At no time were the indices of

TABLE 2.—SERIAL CHANGES IN CARDIAC OUTPUT AND CONTRACTILITY DURING POSTBURN RESUSCITATION*

	TIME PERIOD (HR)			NORMAL VALUES
INDEX	0–12	12–24	24–28	
ECHO CI (L/min/m²)	3.11 ± .25†	2.75 ± .25†	4.03 ± .40	3.40 ± .04
EDVI (ml/m²)	43 ± 3†	36 ± 4†	51 ± 4	60 ± 3
V_{cf} (circ/sec)	1.72 ± .08†	1.68 ± .10†	1.70 ± .09†	1.22 ± .06
EF	0.79 ± .02	0.75 ± .02	0.75 ± .02	0.74 ± .02

*Values are in means ± SEM. CI, cardiac index; EDVI, end-diastolic volume index; V_{cf}, rate of ventricular fiber shortening; EF, ejection fraction.
†$P < .05$ (vs. normal).

myocardial contractility depressed, and the mean velocity of left ventricular internal fiber shortening (V_{cf}) was significantly elevated at all time intervals, indicating a hypercontractile state. These findings implicate intravascular volume deficit as the cause of the decreased cardiac output following thermal injury and provide convincing evidence against the presence of a circulating myocardial depressant factor.

FLUID COMPOSITION AND VOLUME

The importance of sodium-containing fluids in replacing intravascular volume deficits following injury is illustrated by the clinical success of the classic burn resuscitation formulas (Table 3). The independent effects of sodium ion and water on volume restitution following burn injury have been defined in an animal model.[41] When the salt content in replacement solutions was varied over a wide range, 1 mEq of sodium ion produced the same effect as 13 ml of salt-free water in restoring cardiac output by 12 hours after burn. The optimal sodium concentration for burn resuscitation solutions is not known. The limiting factor in sodium composition is hyponatremia or hypernatremia. Since the composition of lost intravascular fluid can best be duplicated by a balanced electrolyte solution, lactated Ringer's solution has been the most widely used formulation for burn resuscitation. Studies in large patient series have demonstrated that fluid losses associated with massive burns can be replaced effectively with large volumes of lactated Ringer's solution without the need for colloid.[38] Hypertonic solutions containing 250 mEq/L were introduced to reduce the volume of fluid infused and attendant tissue edema.[42]

Although the ideal physiologic criteria of resuscitation adequacy remain undefined, numerous clinical studies yield relatively consistent results following the use of hypotonic, isotonic, and hypertonic solutions. As sodium concentration is increased from moderately hypotonic (approximately 100 mEq/L) to moderately hypertonic (250 mEq/L) concentrations, progressively less fluid volume is required for adequate resuscitation.[43] Further, net fluid balance, maximal weight gain, and duration of postresuscitation diuresis are inversely proportional to sodium concentration.[44] No studies have demonstrated the superior efficacy of any sodium concentration in improving

TABLE 3.—Resuscitation Formulas for Adult Burn Patients

COMPONENT	EVANS	PARKLAND	MODIFIED BROOKE	HYPERTONIC
FIRST 24 HOURS				
Lactated Ringer's	· · ·	4 ml/kg/% burn	2/ml/kg/% burn	· · ·
Normal saline	1 ml/kg/% burn	· · ·	· · ·	Volume to maintain urine output at 0.5–1.0 ml/kg/hr
Hypertonic saline	· · ·	· · ·	· · ·	· · ·
Colloid	1 ml/kg/% burn	· · ·	· · ·	· · ·
Sodium-free water	2,000 ml	· · ·	· · ·	· · ·
SECOND 24 HOURS				
Normal saline	½ of first 24-hr requirement	· · ·	· · ·	· · ·
Colloid	½ of first 24-hr requirement	20%–60% of calculated plasma volume	0.3–0.5 ml/kg/% burn	· · ·
Sodium-free water	2,000 ml	Volume to maintain adequate urinary output	Volume to maintain adequate urinary output	Orally up to 3,500 ml

survival. However, the ability of hypertonic solutions to produce less wound edema may be advantageous, particularly in
patients with inhalation injury, circumferential full-thickness
burns of extremities, and intracranial injuries, where massive
fluid accumulation can produce catastrophic complications. The
factor limiting use of hypertonic saline solutions is hypernatremia, and serum sodium concentrations exceeding 160 mEq/L
are associated with oliguria.[45] The success of all these fluid formulations speaks more for the physiologic reserve of the average burned patient than for any specific burn formula.[46]

The role of colloid in tissue fluid loss and in subsequent resuscitation needs remains controversial. Previous studies by
Pruitt et al. in a well-defined group of patients with a mean
burn size of 65% of BSA demonstrated an obligatory plasma
volume loss during the first 24 hours postburn.[36] In these adult
patients with large burns, the calculated rate of plasma loss in
the absence of resuscitation was 4.4 ml/kg/hour. During the
second 24 postburn hours, capillary permeability returned to
normal, with a small calculated net increase in plasma volume
at zero fluid replacement rate. Early animal studies and clinical trials indicated that plasma volume alterations during the
first 24 hours after burn were independent of colloid content of
replacement fluid and that colloid produced a positive effect on
blood volume restoration during the second postburn day.[33, 41]
These observations were qualitatively substantiated by a randomized controlled trial evaluating crystalloid (lactated Ringer's solutions) and colloid (2.5% albumin–lactated Ringer's solution) resuscitation fluids.[40] The repair of the protein leak, at
least in operational terms, appears to occur between 12 and 24
hours after injury, since colloid-containing solutions were more
effective in restoring intravascular volume and cardiac index
to normal at the end of the first 24 hours following injury (Figs
1 and 2). Furthermore, the patients receiving colloid-containing fluid required significantly less volume for adequate resuscitation than the patients receiving the crystalloid solution
(2.98 vs. 3.81 ml/kg/% burn). However, by the end of the second
postburn day, there were no differences between the two treatment groups in terms of fluid volume administered, cardiac
output, and intravascular volume.

The potential advantages of colloid-containing resuscitation
solutions appear to be more than offset by the deleterious ef-

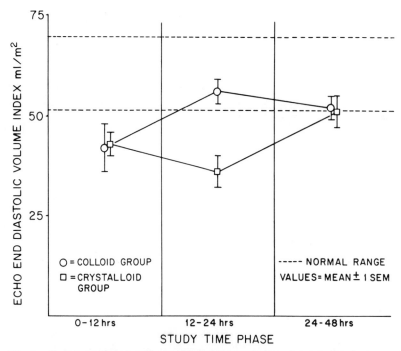

Fig 1.—Serial changes in left ventricular end-diastolic volume index during post-burn resuscitation with colloid and crystalloid solutions.

fects of colloid on the lungs. The level of plasma oncotic pressure does not influence lung water in burned patients.[47, 48] Rather, the administration of colloid in the form of albumin to a series of burned patients was associated with severe pulmonary edema. Administered albumin appears to leak rapidly into the pulmonary interstitium through injured capillaries and to produce a subtraction effect on the intravascular compartment.[49] In animal models of other hypovolemic states, resuscitation with colloid-containing fluid has been associated with a greater increase in lung water than occurred with crystalloid fluid.[50, 51] Direct evidence of the deleterious effects of colloid-containing burn resuscitation solutions on pulmonary physiology was defined in the above-mentioned controlled clinical trial of fluid composition.[40] Lung water in colloid-treated patients increased significantly during the first burn week (Fig 3). By contrast, lung water in the crystalloid-treated patients

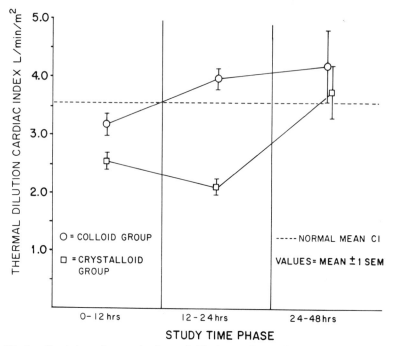

Fig 2.—Postinjury changes in thermal dilution cardiac index. Note that the colloid solution restores total body blood flow more promptly but that both colloid and crystalloid solutions are equally effective by the end of the resuscitation phase.

did not change significantly during the 7-day study. Furthermore, later pulmonary complications and mortality appeared to be higher in the colloid-treated group (Table 4).

STRATEGY OF FLUID ADMINISTRATION

The various resuscitation formulas used for estimating fluid requirements of burned patients are outlined in Table 3. The actual rate of infusion is guided by the patient's physiologic response to the administered fluid, not by formula calculations. Most burned patients can be managed successfully by monitoring urinary output, mental status, and vital signs. Urinary output is the most accessible and effective guideline to adequate resuscitation. Hourly rates of 30–60 ml in adults and 1 ml/kg of body weight in children weighing less than 30 kg indicate adequate fluid replacement and organ perfusion in most situ-

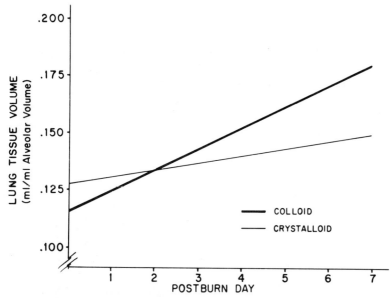

Fig 3.—Effect of resuscitation fluid composition on lung water. While lung water in patients receiving crystalloid solutions remained unchanged during the first postburn week, lung water in patients receiving colloid solutions progressively increased.

ations. Oliguria nearly always indicates underresuscitation. Confusion and anxiety often indicate persistent hypovolemia, and these symptoms usually abate with added volume loading. Heart rate is a reliable indicator of volume status in patients without preexisting heart disease. Generally, pulse rate rises in parallel with the fall in cardiac output and intravascular volume. In adults, rates exceeding 140 beats per minute indicate inadequate resuscitation, while rates of 110–130 beats per minute are associated with satisfactory volume restitution and

TABLE 4.—Patient Outcome in Randomized
Trial Comparing Colloid and Crystalloid
Resuscitation of Burned Patients

	COLLOID	CRYSTALLOID
Total no. of patients	25	25
Roentgenographic pulmonary edema by PBD 7	5	1
Deaths	11	3

organ perfusion. Measurement of arterial blood pressure is difficult and unreliable, even with an ultrasonic flowmeter. Patients not responding to standard resuscitation therapy and those with chronic medical diseases or associated injuries require invasive monitoring of arterial pressure, pulmonary capillary wedge pressure, and cardiac output.

Control of Wound Infection

BURN WOUND INFECTION

Thermal injury causes coagulation necrosis of the epidermis and of varying levels of the dermis and subcutaneous tissue. The burn wound often is not of uniform depth. A deeper central zone of necrosis usually is surrounded by concentric rings of progressively less severe injury.[52] In the regions of capillary stasis, potentially salvageable skin may undergo full-thickness necrosis if poor tissue perfusion or bacterial infection supervenes. Meticulous patient care can limit the extent of tissue loss. Once necrosis occurs, the wound is essentially avascular, which prevents effective delivery of systemic antibiotics if infection occurs. Damage to the cutaneous barrier allows bacterial penetration into viable tissue and subsequent infection.

The pattern of burn wound infection has changed over the past several decades and may be related to the proliferation of broad-spectrum antibiotics. Before the availability of penicillin, streptococci and staphylococci were the predominant organisms. By the late 1950s, gram-negative bacteria, primarily *Pseudomonas* species, emerged as the dominant organisms causing fatal wound infections in burned patients. In general, all wounds become contaminated soon after injury with either the patient's endogenous flora or with the resident organisms in the treatment facility. Microbial species colonize the surface of the wound and may penetrate the avascular eschar. This event is without clinical significance. Bacterial proliferation may occur beneath the eschar at the viable-nonviable interface, leading to subeschar suppuration and separation of the eschar. In a few patients, microorganisms may breach this barrier and invade the underlying viable tissue, producing systemic sepsis. In 1961 Rabin et al. identified the burn wound as a portal for bacterial entry into the blood.[53] *Pseudomonas aeruginosa* produces the prototypical lesion of invasive burn wound sepsis, and the histologic characteristics of such infections have been carefully studied.[54–56] The essential pathologic feature of burn wound sepsis is invasion by the organism into viable tissue. The organisms then spread to the perivascular structures and directly invade the vessel wall, causing a capillaritis with subsequent vascular occlusion. Hemorrhagic necrosis of the surrounding tissue follows, and later the organisms gain entry into the bloodstream to produce metastatic lesions. In unburned tissue, metastatic *P. aeruginosa* results in ecthyma gangrenosum. Depending on the infecting agent, other histologic presentations may occur.

Any organism capable of invading tissue can produce burn wound sepsis. The predominant organism causing wound infection varies with each burn treatment facility. These facilities experience cyclical variations in the pattern of major offending organisms. *Providencia stuartii* almost entirely replaced all other organisms during a 3-year period at the U.S. Army Institute of Surgical Research.[57] A recent evaluation of burn wound infection at the Institute of Surgical Research revealed a more diverse pattern of infection.[58] Although gram-negative bacteria predominated, a large number of patients were invaded by fungi or multiple organisms (Table 5). Burn wound infection could be focal, multifocal, or generalized. Clinically, the likelihood of septicemia appears to increase as the area of burn wound involvement increases. Septicemia caused by an infected burn wound is less frequent in patients with focal invasion (51% in this series) and multifocal invasion involving less than 20% of BSA. Generalized burn wound invasion is consid-

TABLE 5.—MICROORGANISMS CAUSING
BURN WOUND INVASION

ORGANISMS	NO. OF CASES*
Staphylococcus	1
Pseudomonas	44
Other gram-negative bacteria	16
Mixed bacteria	8
Mycotic	18
Bacteria/mycotic	10
Total	97

*Of 763 admissions.

ered to be present when the infection involves areas exceeding 20% of BSA and is associated with a high frequency of septicemia (91% in this series). Since the introduction of effective topical chemotherapy, fungal burn wound infection has increased and primarily involves highly invasive *Phycomycetes* and *Aspergillus* species.[59] *Candida,* while frequently colonizing the wound surface, has little invasive potential and rarely causes burn wound sepsis.[60, 61] Viral infection, usually with herpesvirus, commonly affects partial-thickness wounds and are of clinical significance only when causing visceral lesions.[62]

MONITORING WOUND INFECTION

Certain groups of patients, e.g., children and those with burns larger than 30% of BSA or with multisystem organ failure, are more likely to develop invasive infection of the burn wound. The wounds of all burned patients should be examined once daily, and more often if systemic signs of sepsis are present. These signs include hypothermia, altered mental status, glucose intolerance, ileus, and oliguria. Burn wound infection is indicated by conversion of a partial-thickness burn to full-thickness necrosis, dark brown or violaceous discoloration of the wound, rapid eschar separation, hemorrhage into the subeschar tissue, and violaceous edema of unburned skin at the wound margins. The peripheral hemorrhagic infarcts of ecthyma gangrenosum are specific for *Pseudomonas* wound infection. The definitive diagnosis of burn wound infection can be made only by wound biopsy. Quantitative surface swab cultures are inaccurate and misleading.[63]

The burn wound biopsy is the only reliable method for accurately establishing the diagnosis of burn wound invasion.[64] The wound should be prepared by mechanical cleansing. Antibacterial solutions and organic solvents should not be used, since these agents may destroy bacteria in the biopsy sample, producing a false negative result. The biopsy should be sufficiently large so that portions can be evaluated by histologic and microbiologic methods. A 500-mg wedge-shaped specimen usually is adequate. It must include not only the lesion-bearing eschar but also underlying or adjacent viable tissue in order to confirm the presence of microbial invasion. Half of the specimen is placed in 10% Formalin and subsequently processed by rapid, not frozen, techniques. Bacteria are identified by Gram stain or hematoxylin-eosin stain and fungi by PAS stain. Such processing can be completed in 3–4 hours. The findings are graded on the basis of microbial involvement, and the single most important sign of burn wound infection is the presence of microbial organisms in unburned tissue (Table 6). The remainder of the biopsy sample is sent to the microbiology laboratory for quantitative culture and for antimicrobial sensitivities. The recovery of more than 10^5 organisms per gram of tissue is highly suggestive of, but not diagnostic of, burn wound infection. Inappropriate selection of biopsy site in separated eschar and failure to include viable tissue may suggest infection when none exists. Similarly, lower counts may accompany histologically confirmed invasion and associated septicemia.[65]

TOPICAL ANTIMICROBIAL CHEMOTHERAPY

Prior to the introduction of effective topical antimicrobial agents, up to 60% of deaths in specialized burn treatment facilities were caused by burn wound sepsis.[3] Each of the three agents with proved effectiveness has a wide spectrum of activity, is applied topically to the burn wound, and has its own peculiar advantages and disadvantages (Table 7).[66–68] All appear to be equally effective in controlling burn wound infection when applied early before heavy colonization has occurred. Only mafenide acetate is able to penetrate the eschar, and it is the only agent capable of suppressing dense bacterial proliferation beneath the eschar surface. Mafenide is especially effec-

TABLE 6.—CLASSIFICATION OF BURN WOUND INFECTION
BY HISTOLOGIC GRADE

Contamination (occasional organism on surface of wound).
Surface colonization (heavy growth limited to wound surface).
Partial penetration (organisms within eschar but not at deep margin).
Complete penetration (organisms identified at deep margin of eschar).
Subeschar space infection (proliferation of microorganisms at viable-nonviable tissue interface).
Invasive infection (microorganisms identified in viable tissue):
  A. Focal microinvasion (early focus in viable tissue).
  B. Multifocal or generalized invasion (extensive spread of microorganisms into viable tissue).
  C. Microvascular involvement (organisms invading blood vessels, making hematogenous spread likely).

TABLE 7.—TOPICAL ANTIMICROBIAL AGENTS FOR BURN WOUND CARE

DESCRIPTION	MAFENIDE ACETATE	SILVER SULFADIAZINE	SILVER NITRATE
Method of use	Exposure	Exposure or single layer dressings	Multilayer occlusive dressings
Composition	11.1% active agent in water-miscible base	1.0% active agent in water-miscible base	0.5% agent in aqueous solution
Advantages	Penetrates eschar; wound readily examined; wide antibacterial spectrum; allows full joint motion and treatment of associated injuries; no gram-negative bacterial resistance; easy to apply	Painless; wound readily examined if used without dressings; no systemic toxicity; allows full joint motion and treatment of associated injuries; easy to apply	No hypersensitivity; painless; no antibacterial resistance; wide spectrum
Disadvantages	Bacteriostatic; painful on 2d-degree burns; delayed eschar separation; hypersensitivity in 7% of patients; carbonic anhydrase inhibition with bicarbonate diuresis	Bacteriostatic; poor penetration into eschar; hypersensitivity (infrequent); gram-negative bacterial resistance; delayed eschar separation; bone marrow suppression of granulocytic series	Bacteriostatic; active only at burn wound surface; must be used early after injury; difficult to use; loss of Na^+, K^+, Cl^-, and Ca^{++} through eschar; dressings inhibit joint mobility and discolor environment and unburned skin; inactive against clostridia

tive in suppressing clostridia. The main disadvantage of mafenide acetate is its strong carbonic anhydrase inhibition, which interferes with renal buffering mechanisms. Bicarbonate is wasted, chloride is retained, and the resulting hyperchloremia is compensated for by an increase in ventilation and subsequent respiratory alkalosis.[69]

The primary disadvantages of silver sulfadiazine are its lack of eschar penetration and the development of bacterial resistance to its antibacterial actions. If bacterial density in the wound increases while silver sulfadiazine is being used, the agent must be discontinued and mafenide acetate, which can penetrate the eschar, substituted. Of greater concern is the increasing development of gram-negative bacterial resistance to this agent.[70, 71] The mode of resistance in some facilities is a transferable, multiple antibiotic–resistant plasmid with selective sulfonamide resistance.[72] The use of silver sulfadiazine in these situations can lead to the selection of organisms which are resistant to all clinically available antibiotics. Silver nitrate must be used after injury, before bacteria have proliferated on the wound. Although gram-positive organisms are slightly less susceptible to silver nitrate, true resistance does not develop. Its most serious disadvantages are the associated electrolyte imbalances, which are common, and methemoglobinemia formation, which is unusual. Methemoglobin may form in patients whose burns are colonized by nitrate-reducing bacteria.[73] No other agents have demonstrated clinical efficacy in clinical trials of topical chemoprophylaxis of burn wounds.

SUBESCHAR CLYSIS

Although topical chemotherapeutic agents have significantly reduced the incidence of burn wound sepsis, this complication. continues to be a major cause of mortality in patients with large burns. Once generalized burn wound sepsis has developed, the probability of survival is less than 10%.[58] Subeschar infusion of antibiotics has been proposed to prevent or treat wound invasion in burn wounds that escape topical chemotherapeutic control.[74]

This therapeutic modality has been systematically examined in an established animal model of burn wound infection and subsequently in burned patients. In a strain of *P. aeruginosa*

(SRU 12-4-4) which predictably produces lethal burn wound sepsis, a range of antibiotics and routes of administration were evaluated.[75] This organism was selected because *Pseudomonas* wound infection remains the major wound-related source of sepsis. The organisms were sensitive by standard tube dilution techniques to carbenicillin, colistimethate, gentamicin, and neomycin. The semisynthetic penicillins, represented in this study by carbenicillin, when injected beneath the infected eschar, resulted in universal survival. Subcutaneous injection of carbenicillin at a site distant to the burn also eradicated burn wound sepsis, although proportionately higher doses were required. IV or intraperitoneal injection of carbenicillin was without effect. Likewise, all animals receiving colistimethate, gentamicin, and neomycin died. Unlike the aminoglycosides, colistimethate, and neomycin, the penicillins are highly diffusible in tissue. The introduction of carbenicillin by the subeschar and subcutaneous routes appears to provide a depot from which sustained blood levels are maintained. Importantly, this study demonstrated that the prospective selection of an effective antibiotic for subeschar therapy cannot be determined by in vitro sensitivity testing.

The effectiveness of subeschar clysis was demonstrated in a clinical series of 19 consecutive patients who developed burn wound infection over a 2-year period.[65] All patients had histologically proved burn wound invasion and were subsequently treated with subeschar clysis of carbenicillin. The clinical effectiveness of subeschar treatment is indicated in Table 8. Five of 19 patients (26%) survived and were discharged from the hospital. Five additional patients died later without evidence of residual burn wound infection. Altogether, subeschar clysis eradicated burn wound invasion in 53% of treated patients.

Subeschar clysis is best utilized as adjunctive therapy in preparation of patients for eschar excision or as primary treatment for patients who are too unstable hemodynamically to tol-

TABLE 8.—CLINICAL OUTCOME FOLLOWING
SUBESCHAR CLYSIS

OUTCOME	NO. OF PTS.
Survivors	5
Patients dying without wound infection	5
Patients dying with wound infection	9

erate surgical intervention. Once the diagnosis of bacterial burn wound invasion is confirmed, topical therapy is changed to mafenide acetate, which is capable of penetrating into underlying viable tissue. Appropriate systemic antibiotics are instituted, usually an aminoglycoside plus a semisynthetic penicillin for control of gram-negative bacteria and an antibiotic effective against gram-positive bacteria. The invaded burn wound is treated directly by subeschar clysis of the semisynthetic penicillin. Even when mycotic burn wound invasion has occurred, subeschar clysis should be utilized since mixed mycotic/bacterial wound infection occurs in a large proportion of these patients. Although focal infection may be totally eradicated by these interventions, excision of the infected wound is the definitive therapy of burn wound invasion. If localized infection is treated only by antimicrobial agents, the successful eradication of the invaded focus must be verified by biopsy and histologic examination. Generalized wound involvement in stable patients should be treated by surgical excision. The wound should be covered immediately with biologic dressings.

Wound Closure

WOUND PREPARATION

Traditional burn wound care involves the gradual removal of nonviable eschar by debridement at the time of the daily wound cleansing procedure. Topical chemotherapy is employed to control wound infection until the defect is ready for autografting. Viable cutaneous allograph is a valuable adjunct in controlling microbial density, reducing evaporative water loss, debriding nonviable elements, and preparing the wound bed for autografting.[76] Such an approach usually requires in excess of 3 weeks to prepare the burn wound closure. Early excision and grafting recently has been advocated to shorten duration of illness and to decrease the mortality associated with a massive burn wound. Nonrandomized, retrospective studies suggest that early excisional therapy may decrease length of hospital stay and mortality in children.[77, 78] Most studies indicate that early surgical excision does not improve survival, although duration of hospital stay appears to be significantly reduced for patients with burns less than 20% of BSA.[6, 79-81] Furthermore, early excision and resurfacing of specialized areas, such as the hands, does not facilitate functional recovery.[7] The limiting factors in early surgical therapy are large blood losses, the pulmonary effects of anesthesia and operation, and the unavailability of sufficient autograft in patients with large burns.

SYNTHETIC WOUND DRESSINGS

Numerous dressings have been utilized to accelerate the healing of partial-thickness injuries. Improved healing would decrease the intensity of the physiologic response to injury, reduce the likelihood of infection and conversion to full-thickness injury, and increase the availability of donor sites in patients with massive burns. Fine mesh gauze is the standard against which all other dressings are compared; donor sites covered with this material heal in approximately 2 weeks.[82] Silicone polymer membranes have been the most widely utilized because of their permeability to water vapor.[83] Recently, polyurethane and polyvinyl chloride polymers have been introduced, all of which have as ideal properties water permeability, elasticity and variable degrees of adherence to the wound. One composite skin substitute, a silicone polymer laminated to a nylon mesh, apparently can be used for both partial- and full-thickness defects, but infection is a major liability when used with the latter wounds.[84] A drawback to dressings applied as a foam, particularly polyurethane, appears to be incorporation of the agent into the cells of the healing wound and subsequent foreign body giant cell reaction.[85] Most of these dressings have been evaluated primarily on donor sites. All reduce wound pain when compared with fine mesh gauze, and some appear to reduce moderately the time to healing. However, studies of this latter advantage are less than rigorous because of variability of donor site depth and lack of histologic quantification of completeness of healing.[86]

In an apparent departure from desired properties of a wound covering, a gas-impermeable dressing employing a hydrocolloid polymer complex has been demonstrated in a well-designed clinical trial to significantly promote partial thickness wound healing and patient comfort.[87] Rate of healing was assayed by wound biopsy on the seventh postoperative day. Pain perception was measured by a blinded observer using both categorical and visual analogue scales. At the time of biopsy, 93% of wounds treated with the hydrocolloid dressing were completely reepithelialized, compared with only 7% of wounds covered with fine mesh gauze. Pain perception likewise was significantly reduced. This study suggests that synthetic wound dressings may justify their greater expense, and serves as a model for evaluation of all similar dressings.

ARTIFICIAL SKIN SUBSTITUTES

The major advance in burn wound closure has been the development of skin substitutes which potentially can be incorporated directly into the healing wound. The two major elements of an artificial skin are the epidermal surface and the underlying matrix on which to support the surface cell layers. Independent research efforts are currently developing each of these components.

The matrix support structure has received substantial laboratory and clinical evaluation. Bell et al. have developed a relatively unstructured collagen gel which is seeded with cultured fibroblasts to serve as a dermal matrix.[88] This dermal lattice can then be covered with epidermal cells. Yannus, Burke, et al. have developed a bilayer polymeric membrane for the closure of full-thickness wounds. The membrane consists of a top layer of silicone elastomer and a bottom layer of a well-structured collagen matrix.[89] The ability of this membrane to be incorporated as a neodermis is exquisitely dependent on average molecular weight between covalent crosslinks, ratio of collagen to glycosaminoglycan, and pore structure. Following grafting, the dermal lattice is populated by fibroblasts and blood vessels from the wound bed. Various stages of this bilayer membrane are utilized with seeded epidermal cells or with very thin split-thickness skin following removal of the silicone layer.

This latter technique has been employed successfully to cover up to 60% of BSA following early excision in massively burned patients.[90] The artificial dermis effectively closes the wound. The Silastic membrane has been left in place for up to 6 weeks while limited donor sites were being repeatedly reharvested. Following removal of the Silastic membrane, the exposed dermal lattice is covered with 0.004-inch-thick autoepidermal grafts. These donor sites heal within a few days. Long-term cosmetic and functional results are reported to be good to excellent.

The epidermal component has been the focus of separate investigations. Normal human epidermal keratinocytes suitable for wound resurfacing can be grown in a defined medium.[91] Autologous cultured cells without a supportive dermal matrix have been grafted onto full-thickness wound beds.[92] These grafts of cultured epithelium survived in vivo and acquired anatomical characteristics similar to those observed with healed autografts. The major limitation to this approach is the requirement of autologous cells in order to avoid graft rejection. Tissue must be harvested from the burned patient for growth in tissue culture into sheets of skin. These techniques are time consuming and sufficient cultured skin for wound closure is not available for several weeks after injury.

A major innovation in wound resurfacing has been the recent development of techniques for growing human epidermal cells in culture with loss of HLA-DR antigen expression.[93] These cells no longer stimulate allogeneic lymphocytes, suggesting that such tissue would be immunologically unrecognizable

Fig 4.—Histologic biopsy section obtained 2 weeks following burn wound closure with cultural epidermal allograft. (Courtesy of Dr. J.M. Hefton).

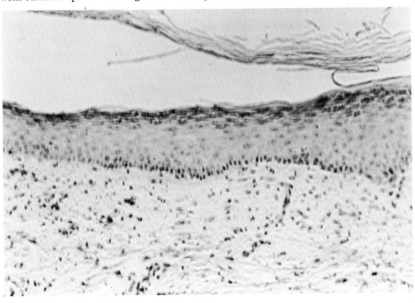

when grafted onto an unrelated recipient.[94] The clinical utility of allografts of cultured epidermal cells was evaluated in three burned patients with tangentially excised deep dermal burns.[95] Such wounds ordinarily would be covered with split-thickness skin. The burn wounds closed with cultured allografts healed within three days and remained healthy for 9 months of observations (Fig 4). Typing of the healed wound with specific donor and recipient markers is needed to confirm the actual incorporation of unrelated tissue into the host, and a suitable dermal matrix probably will be required for utilizing epidermal allografts on full-thickness wounds. Nevertheless, sheets of epidermal allografts can be grown in large quantities and stored for immediate use, and even in the present state appear to be efficacious for the closure of many excised wounds.

REFERENCES

1. Editorial. *National Burn Information Exchange Newsletter* 2:1, 1983.
2. Cope O., Moore F.D.: The redistribution of body water in the fluid therapy of the burned patient. *Ann. Surg.* 126:1013, 1947.
3. Pruitt B.A. Jr., O'Neill J.A., Moncrief J.A., et al.: Successful control of burn wound sepsis. *JAMA* 203:1054, 1968.
4. Bull J.P., Squire J.R.: A study of mortality in a burns unit. *Ann. Surg.* 130:160, 1949.
5. Pruitt B.A. Jr., Tumbusch W.T., Mason A.D. Jr., et al.: Mortality in 1,100 consecutive burns treated at a burns unit. *Ann. Surg.* 159:396, 1964.
6. Curreri P.W., Luterman A., Braun D.W. Jr., et al.: Burn injury: Analysis of survival and hospitalization time for 937 patients. *Ann. Surg.* 192:472, 1980.
7. Goodwin C.W., Maguire M.S., McManus W.F., et al.: Prospective study of burn wound excision of the hands. *J. Trauma* 23:510, 1983.
8. Moylan J.A., Pruitt B.A. Jr.: Aeromedical transportation. *JAMA* 224:1271, 1973.
9. Treat R.C., Sirinek K.R., Levine B.A., et al.: Air evacuation of thermally injured patients: Principles of treatments and results. *J. Trauma* 20:275, 1980.
10. Pruitt B.A. Jr., McManus W.F., Kim S.H., et al.: Diagnosis and treatment of intravenous cannula related sepsis in burn patients. *Ann. Surg.* 191:546, 1980.
11. Sasaki T.M., Panke T.W., Dorethy J.F., et al.: The relationship of central venous and pulmonary artery catheter position to acute right-sided endocarditis in severe thermal injury. *J. Trauma* 19:740, 1979.
12. Baskin T.W., Rosenthal A., Pruitt B.A. Jr.: Acute bacterial endocarditis: A silent source of sepsis in the burned patient. *Ann. Surg.* 184:618, 1976.
13. Cohn I. Jr., Bornside G.H.: Infections, in Schwartz S.I., Shires G.T., Spencer F.C., et al.: (eds.): *Principles of Surgery*. New York, McGraw-Hill Book Co., 1984, p. 188.

14. Czaja A.J., McAlhany J.C., Pruitt B.A. Jr.: Acute gastroduodenal disease after thermal injury: An endoscopic evaluation of incidence and natural history. *N. Engl. J. Med.* 291:925, 1974.
15. Czaja A.J., McAlhany J.C., Pruitt B.A. Jr.: Acute duodenitis and duodenal ulceration after burns: Clinical and pathological characteristics. *JAMA* 232:621, 1975.
16. Czaja A.J., McAlhany J.C., Pruitt B.A. Jr.: Acute gastric disease after cutaneous thermal injury. *Arch. Surg.* 110:600, 1975.
17. McAlhany J.C. Jr., Czaja A.J., Pruitt B.A. Jr.: Antacid control of complications from acute gastroduodenal disease after burns. *J. Trauma* 16:645, 1976.
18. McElwee H.P., Sirinek K.R., Levine B.A.: Cimetidine affords protection equal to antacids in prevention of stress ulceration following thermal injury. *Surgery* 86:620, 1979.
19. Agee R.N., Long J.M. III, Hunt J.L., et al.: Use of [133]xenon in early diagnosis of inhalation injury. *J. Trauma* 16:218, 1976.
20. Moylan J.A., Adib K., Burnbaum M.: Fiberoptic bronchoscopy following thermal injury. *Surg. Gynecol. Obstet.* 140:541, 1975.
21. Moylan J.A., Wilmore D.W., Mouton D.E., et al.: Early diagnosis of inhalation injury using [133]xenon lung scan. *Ann. Surg.* 176:477, 1972.
22. Petroff P.A., Hander E.W., Clayton W.H., et al.: Pulmonary function studies after smoke inhalation. *Am. J. Surg.* 132:346, 1976.
23. Welch G.W., Lull R.J., Petroff P.A., et al.: The use of steroids in inhalation injury. *Surg. Gynecol. Obstet.* 145:539, 1977.
24. Levine B.A., Petroff P.A., Slade C.L., et al.: Prospective trials of dexamethasone and aerosolized gentamicin in the burned patient. *J. Trauma* 18:188, 1978.
25. Moylan J.A., Chan C.K.: Inhalation injury—an increasing problem. *Ann. Surg.* 188:34, 1978.
26. Pruitt B.A. Jr., Bowling J.A., Moncrief J.A.: Escharotomy in early burn care. *Arch. Surg.* 96:502, 1968.
27. Moylan J.A., Inge W.W., Pruitt B.A. Jr.: Circulatory changes following circumferential extremity burns evaluated by the ultrasonic flowmeter: Analysis of 60 thermally injured limbs. *J. Trauma* 11:763, 1971.
28. Clayton J.M., Russell H.E., Hartford C.E., et al.: Sequential circulatory changes in the circumferentially burned limb. *Ann. Surg.* 185:391, 1977.
29. Hunt J.L., Sato R.M., Baxter C.R.: Acute electric burns: Current diagnosis and therapeutic approaches to management. *Arch. Surg.* 115:434, 1980.
30. Arturson G.: Pathophysiological aspects of the burn syndrome. *Acta. Chir. Scand. Suppl.* 274:1, 1961.
31. Demling R.H., Kramer G., Harns B.: Role of thermal injury-induced hypoproteinemia in burned and nonburned tissue. *Surgery* 95:136, 1984.
32. Blalock A.: Trauma to intestines: The importance of the local loss of fluid in the production of low blood pressure. *Arch. Surg.* 22:314, 1931.
33. Baxter C.R.: Fluid volume and electrolyte changes of the early postburn period. *Clin. Past. Surg.* 1:693, 1974.
34. Topley E., Jackson D.M., Cason J.S., et al.: Assessment of red cell loss in the first two days after severe burns. *Ann. Surg.* 155:581, 1962.

35. Asch M.J., Meserol P.M., Mason A.D. Jr., et al.: Regional blood flow in the burned anesthetized dog. *Surg. Forum* 22:55, 1971.
36. Pruitt B.A. Jr., Mason A.D. Jr., Moncrief J.A.: Hemodynamic changes in the early postburn patient: The influence of fluid administration and of a vasodilator (Hydralazine). *J. Trauma* 11:36, 1971.
37. Baxter C.R., Cook W.A., Shires G.T.: Serum myocardial depressant factor of burn shock. *Surg. Forum* 17:1, 1966.
38. Baxter C.R., Shires G.T.: Physiological response to crystalloid resuscitation of severe burns. *Ann. NY Acad. Sci.* 150:874, 1968.
39. Shoemaker W.C., Vladeck B.C., Bassin R., et al.: Burn pathophysiology in man: I. Sequential hemodynamic alterations. *J. Surg. Res.* 14:64, 1973.
40. Goodwin C.W., Dorethy J., Lam V., et al.: Randomized trial of efficacy of crystalloid and colloid resuscitation on hemodynamic response and lung water following thermal injury. *Ann. Surg.* 197:520, 1983.
41. Moylan J.A., Mason D.A. Jr., Rogers P.W., et al.: Postburn shock: A critical evaluation of resuscitation. *J. Trauma* 13:354, 1973.
42. Monafo W.W., Chuntrasakul C., Ayvazian V.H.: Hypertonic sodium solutions in the treatment of burn shock. *Am. J. Surg.* 126:778, 1973.
43. Monafo W.W., Halverson J.D., Schechtman K.: The role of concentrated sodium solutions in the resuscitation of patients with severe burns. *Surgery* 95:129, 1984.
44. Bowser B.H., Caldwell F.T.: The effects of resuscitation with hypertonic vs. hypotonic vs. colloid on wound and urine fluid and electrolyte losses in severely burned children. *J. Trauma* 23:916, 1983.
45. Shimazaki S., Yosioka T., Tanaka N., et al.: Body fluid changes during hypertonic saline solution therapy for burn shock. *J. Trauma* 17:38, 1977.
46. Pruitt B.A. Jr.: Fluid resuscitation for extensively burned patients. *J. Trauma Suppl.* 21:690, 1981.
47. Lam V., Goodwin C.W., Treat R.C., et al.: Does pulmonary extravascular water vary with colloid oncotic pressure after burn injury? *Am. Rev. Respir. Dis.* 119:139, 1979.
48. Tranbaugh R.F., Lewis F.R., Christnsen J.M., et al.: Lung water after thermal injury: The effect of crystalloid resuscitation and sepsis. *Ann. Surg.* 192:479, 1980.
49. Goodwin C.W., Long J.M., Mason A.D. Jr., et al.: Paradoxical effect of hyperoncotic albumin in acutely burned children. *J. Trauma* 21:63, 1981.
50. Holcroft J.W., Trunkey D.D.: Extravascular lung water following hemorrhagic shock in the baboon: Comparison between resuscitation with Ringer's lactate and Plasmanate. *Ann. Surg.* 180:408, 1974.
51. Schloerb P.R., Hunt P.T., Plummer J.A., et al.: Pulmonary edema after replacement of blood loss by electrolyte solutions. *Surg. Gynecol. Obstet.* 135:893, 1972.
52. Order S.E., Mason A.D. Jr., Walker H.L., et al.: The pathogenesis of second and third degree burns and conversion to full thickness injury. *Surg. Gynecol. Obstet.* 120:983, 1965.
53. Rabin E.R., Graber C.O., Vogel E.H., et al.: Fatal *Pseudomonas* infection

in burned patients: A clinical, bacteriologic, and anatomic study. *N. Engl. J. Med.* 265:1225, 1961.

54. Teplitz C.: Pathogenesis of *Pseudomonas* vasculitis and septic lesions. *Arch. Pathol.* 80:297, 1965.
55. Teplitz C., Davis D., Walker H.L., et al.: *Pseudomonas* burn wound sepsis. *J. Surg. Res.* 4:200, 1964.
56. Teplitz C., Davis D., Walker H.L.: *Pseudomonas* burn wound sepsis: II. Hematogenous infection at the junction of the burn wound and the unburned hypodermis. *J. Surg. Res.* 4:217, 1964.
57. Curreri P.W., Bruck H.M., Lindberg R.B., et al.: *Providencia stuartii* sepsis: A new challenge in the treatment of thermal injury. *Ann. Surg.* 177:133, 1973.
58. McManus W.F., Goodwin C.W., Mason A.D. Jr., et al.: Burn wound infection. *J. Trauma* 21:753, 1981.
59. Nash G., Foley F.D., Goodwin M.N. Jr., et al.: Fungal burn wound infection. *JAMA* 215:1664, 1971.
60. Bruck H.M., Nash G., Stein J.M., et al.: Studies on the occurrence and significance of yeasts and fungi in the burn wound. *Ann. Surg.* 176:108, 1972.
61. Nash G., Foley F.D., Pruitt B.A. Jr.: *Candida* burn wound invasion: A cause of systemic candidasis. *Arch. Pathol.* 90:75, 1970.
62. Foley F.D., Greenwald K.A., Nash G., et al.: Herpesvirus infection in burned patients. *N. Engl. J. Med.* 282:652, 1970.
63. Pruitt B.A. Jr.: The burn patient: II. Later care and complications of thermal injury. *Curr. Probl. Surg.* 16:17, 1979.
64. Pruitt B.A. Jr., Foley F.D.: The use of biopsies in burn care. *Surgery* 73:887, 1973.
65. McManus W.F., Goodwin C.W., Pruitt B.A. Jr.: Subeschar treatment of burn wound infection. *Arch. Surg.* 118:291, 1983.
66. Moncrief J.A., Lindberg R.B., Switzer W.E., et al.: The use of topical sulfonamide in the control of burn wound sepsis. *J. Trauma* 6:407, 1966.
67. Moyer C.A., Brentano L., Gravens D.L., et al.: Treatment of large human burns with 0.5 percent silver nitrate solution. *Arch. Surg.* 90:812, 1965.
68. Fox C.L. Jr., Rappole B.W., Stanford W.: Control of *Pseudomonas* infection in burns by silver sulfadiazine. *Surg. Gynecol. Obstet.* 128:1021, 1969.
69. Asch M.J., White M.G., Pruitt B.A. Jr.: Acid-base changes associated with topical Sulfamylon therapy: Retrospective study of 100 burn patients. *Ann. Surg.* 172:946, 1970.
70. Bridges K., Lowbury F.J.L.: Drug resistance in relation to use of silver sulfadiazine cream in a burns unit. *J. Clin. Pathol.* 30:160, 1977.
71. Lowbury E.J.L., Babb J.R., Bridges K., et al.: Topical chemoprophylaxis with silver sulfadiazine, silver nitrate, and chlorhexidine creams: Emergence of sulfonamide-resistant gram negative bacilli. *Br. Med. J.* 1:493, 1976.
72. McManus A.T., Denton C.L., Mason A.D. Jr.: Mechanism of in vitro sensitivity to sulfadiazine silver. *Arch. Surg.* 118:161, 1983.
73. Ternberg J.L., Luce E.: Methemoglobinemia: A complication of silver nitrate treatment of burns. *Surgery* 63:328, 1968.

74. Baxter C.R., Curreri P.W., Marvin J.A.: The control of burn wound sepsis by the use of quantitative bacteriologic studies and subeschar clysis of antibiotics. *Surg. Clin. North Am.* 53:1509, 1973.
75. McManus W.F., Mason A.D. Jr., Pruitt B.A. Jr.: Subeschar antibiotic infusion in the treatment of burn wound infection. *J. Trauma* 20:1021, 1980.
76. Shuck J.M., Pruitt B.A. Jr., Moncrief J.A.: Homograft for wound coverage: A study in versatility. *Arch. Surg.* 98:472, 1969.
77. Burke J.F., Bondec C.C., Quinby W.C.: Primary burn excision and immediate grafting: A method shortening illness. *J. Trauma* 14:389, 1974.
78. Burke J.F., Quinby W.C., Bondoc C.C.: Primary excision and prompt grafting as routine therapy for the treatment of thermal burns in children. *Surg. Clin. North Am.* 56:477, 1976.
79. Levine B.A., Sirinek K.R., Pruitt B.A. Jr.: Wound excision to facia in burn patients. *Arch. Surg.* 113:403, 1978.
80. Gray D.T., Pine R.W., Hamar J.T., et al.: Early surgical excision vs. conventional therapy in 20–40 percent burns: A comparative study. *Am. J. Surg.* 144:76, 1982.
81. Engrave L.H., Heimback D.M., Reus J.L., et al.: Early excision and grafting vs nonoperative treatment of burns of indeterminant depth: A randomized prospective study. *J. Trauma* 23:1001, 1983.
82. Artz C.P., Bronwell A.W., Sako Y.: The exposure treatment of donor sites. *Am. J. Surg.* 142:248, 1955.
83. Tavis M.J., Thornton J., Danet R., et al.: Current status of skin substitutes. *Surg. Clin. North Am.* 58:1233, 1978.
84. Zachary L., Heggers J.P., Robson M.C., et al.: The use of topical antimicrobials combined with Biobrane in burn wound infections. *J. Trauma* 22:833, 1982.
85. Salisbury R.E., Bevin A.G., Dingeldein G.P., et al.: A clinical and laboratory evaluation of a polyurethane foam. *Arch. Surg.* 114:1188, 1979.
86. James J.H., Watson A.C.: The use of Opsite, a vapour-permeable dressing, on skin graft donor sites. *Br. J. Plast. Surg.* 28:107, 1975.
87. Madden M.R., Finkelstein J.L., Hefton J.M., et al.: Hydrocolloid dressings (HCD) accelerate the healing of partial thickness donor site wounds. *Proc. Am. Burn Assoc.,* 1984, p. 12.
88. Bell E., Erlich H.P., Buttle D.J., et al.: Living tissue formed in vitro and accepted as skin equivalent tissue of full thickness. *Science* 211:1052, 1981.
89. Yannus I.V., Burke J.F., Orgill D.P., et al.: Wound tissue can utilize a polymeric template to synthesize a functional extension of skin. *Science* 215:174, 1982.
90. Burke J.F., Yannas I.V., Quinby W.C., et al.: Successful use of a physiologically acceptable artificial skin in the treatment of extensive burn injury. *Ann. Surg.* 194:413, 1981.
91. Tsao M.C., Walthall B.J., Ham R.G.: Clonal growth of normal human epidermal keratinocytes in a defined medium. *J. Cell Physiol.* 110:219, 1982.
92. O'Connor N.E., Mulliken J.B., Banks-Schegel S., et al.: Grafting of burns

with cultured epithelium prepared from autologous epidermal cells. *Lancet* 1:75, 1981.
93. Eisinger M., Lee J.S., Hefton J.M., et al.: Human epidermal cell cultures: Growth and differentiation in the absence of dermal components and medium supplements. *Proc. Natl. Acad. Sci. USA* 76:5340, 1979.
94. Hefton J.M., Amberson J.G., Biozes D.G., et al.: Human epidermal cells no longer stimulate allogeneic lymphocytes after growth in culture. *J. Invest. Dermatol.* 76:308, 1981.
95. Hefton J.M., Madden M.R., Finkelstein J.L., et al.: Grafting of burn patients with allographs of cultured epidermal cells. *Lancet* 2:4028, 1983.

Implantable Infusion Pumps

HENRY BUCHWALD, M.D., PH.D.
AND THOMAS D. ROHDE, M.S.

Department of Surgery, University of Minnesota, Minneapolis, Minnesota

To be effective, a pharmaceutical agent must be capable of reaching its site of activity in the body and remaining present in concentrations sufficient to achieve the desired therapeutic effect but not sufficient to cause undesirable side effects. While medical science has made great strides during the past 50 years in selecting and modifying the molecular structures and formulations of drugs to optimize their pharmacochemical properties, means were not available, heretofore, to exploit fully drug capabilities on the basis of pharmacokinetic principles. The failure of conventional oral and parenteral drug delivery methods to circumvent many of the obstacles to effective drug action has undoubtedly prevented many existing drugs from reaching their maximum therapeutic potential and has hindered the development of many potentially useful therapeutic agents.

Oral administration of drugs is the method of choice for most physicians, mainly because it is convenient and noninvasive. It does, however, have a number of limitations. In order to avoid destruction and to reach their site of activity in adequate quantity to achieve the desired therapeutic effect, successful oral agents must be, in large part, immune to the effects of gastric acid in the stomach, the enzymes in the intestine (both natural and produced by enteric bacteria), and the catabolic processes of the liver. Additionally, they must be capable of absorption through the intestinal wall. Some drugs that fail to meet these

177

0065–3411/84/0018–0177–0222–$04.00

criteria can be administered parenterally, but whether given by mouth or by injection, few drugs can be maintained at constant serum concentrations using oral or intermittent injection administration methodology. Typically, a high blood level is reached shortly after administration, followed by a gradual decline as the drug is excreted by the kidneys, catabolized by the liver, or removed in gaseous form by the lungs. This peak and valley pattern can be overcome by continuous intravenous (IV) drug delivery, but until the advent of the implantable drug infusion pump, such therapy generally required that the patient be hospitalized. The option for continuous, precisely controlled drug delivery into a variety of body sites in ambulatory subjects became available for widespread use by the medical community in March 1981, when the first implantable infusion pump was approved by the Food and Drug Administration (FDA) for IV delivery of heparin and intra-arterial infusion of 5-fluouroxyuridine (5-FUDR).

Kinds of Implantable Drug Delivery Systems

There are an array of devices that could conceivably be considered under the topic of "implantable pumps." Such devices include implantable pellets and capsules, rate-specified pharmaceuticals, passive implantable infusion devices, and active implantable infusion devices. These categories are reviewed briefly below.

IMPLANTED PELLETS AND CAPSULES

One of the earliest attempts to achieve controlled long-term drug release was through the use of implantable capsules and pellets which are placed under the skin and are slowly dissolved by body fluids and released into the subcutaneous tissues. This technique was introduced in 1937 by Deansley and Parks, who demonstrated that implanted capsules of compressed estrone caused female feather patterns to develop in male capons and remain for periods as long as 3 months.[1] In recent years, macromolecular drugs in powder form are often cast in biocompatible polymeric matrices that slow dissolution of the drug and prolong its effect. A substantial degree of control over the drug release rate can be achieved by shaping the capsule so that an increased area of drug surface becomes available for release as the distance from the release surface increases. Additional control of drug release rate has been achieved by the addition of magnetic beads to the polymeric matrix and stimulating increased drug release by placing an oscillating bar magnet over the casule. Release rate increases of up to 200% have been achieved by this method. The mechanism for this increased drug release rate is not clearly understood but may be caused by the alternate compression and expansion of the flexible passageways in the matrix, thereby squeezing the drug from the capsule.[2]

RATE-SPECIFIED PHARMACEUTICALS

Rate-specified pharmaceuticals are those in which label specifications of drug strength are given as rate, duration, and concentration. Alza Corporation (Palo Alto, Calif.) has been a leader in the development of technology of this type. One of their devices is the Ocusert pilocarpine ocular therapeutic system which is worn beneath the eyelid to minimize the side effects of miosis and myopia that often occur with pilocarpine eye drops.[3] Another rate-specified drug release system is the Progestasert intrauterine progesterone contraceptive system. This is an intrauterine device that utilizes progesterone, which has a half-life of one-half hour, to serve as a contraceptive for a duration of 1 year and also has the beneficial side effect of reducing menstrual blood loss by one half.[2, 4]

One of the first totally implantable rate-controlled infusion devices for the administration of liquid infusates was described by Rose and Nelson in 1955.[5] Their device used osmotic pressure produced by a saturated aqueous solution of Congo red in a partially collapsed rubber bag separated from a second compartment containing water by a semipermeable cellophane membrane. As the water moved into the Congo red solution by osmosis, the rubber bag expanded, expelling the drug from the pump. Later osmotic pump designs developed by Alza Corporation differ from that of Rose and Nelson in that they use water from the cellular environment to produce osmotic pressure rather than having a second water compartment.[6] Using this approach, they developed the simple and inexpensive Alzet Osmotic Minipump that has seen widespread use in animal pharmacologic studies. These devices are readily implantable in laboratory animals as small as mice and provide 2–4 weeks of relatively constant drug delivery.

No attempt has been made, to date, to develop a clinical version of the Alzet pump. The suitability of implantable osmotic devices for clinical use is impaired by their lacking the ability to be refilled. This difficulty is not a problem with the Oros rate-controlled pharmaceutical delivery system, which is designed for oral ingestion. This system resembles a conventional capsule in appearance but is actually a small osmotic pump based on the same technology as the Alzet Minipump. The system contains a core of solid drug, coated with a semipermeable membrane having a single small orifice. Water from the gastrointestinal tract is selectively drawn into the capsule by the osmotic gradient between the gastrointestinal fluid and the drug. Since the capsule's volume cannot expand, the drug flows out of the capsular orifice at the same rate the water moves into the capsule by osmosis. Thus, the drug is released at a relatively constant rate as the drug infusion system moves through the digestive tract.[7] Lack of ability to refill the system is not a hindrance in this case because subsequent capsules can be ingested as the capsules run out of drug or pass out of the alimentary canal.

PASSIVE IMPLANTABLE INFUSION DEVICES

For the purposes of this chapter, passive implantable infusion devices are defined as those that lack an intrinsic power source so that infusion occurs only when energy is supplied from outside the device. Examples of such devices are the Ommaya reservoir, which was designed to provide long-term access to the cerebrospinal fluid, the Levene and Denver shunts for relief of ascites, an externally driven implantable roller pump designed for the treatment of hydrocephalus and ascites, and the Infuse-A-Port, a device for long-term vascular access.

The Ommaya reservoir is a mushroom-shaped capsule designed for connection to an intraventricular or intrathecal catheter. The dome is made of a specially thickened silicone rubber designed to accommodate up to 200 needle punctures without leaking. Thus, fluid can be injected into or removed from the reservoir. It is also compressible and can be used as a simple pump if pressure is exerted on the skin over the capsule.[8]

Use of a peritoneovenous shunt for the treatment of chronic intractable ascites was introduced by Smith and associates in 1962.[9] They connected the peritoneal cavity to the saphenous vein by means of a unidirectional low-pressure Holter valve. By manually squeezing the valve, they were able to drain the coelomic fluid back into the venous circulation. Leveen et al. devised a modified version of this shunt that utilized pressure- or flow-activated one-way valves in place of the Holter valve. To operate the pressure-activated valve, the patient inspires against a resistance of 5 cm H_2O to increase the differential pressure between the peritoneum and the venous circulation.[10] Currently, the Storz Denver Peritoneo-Venous Shunt (manufactured by Denver Biomaterials, Inc.; sold by Storz Instrument Co., St. Louis, Missouri) is also available. It utilizes two one-way valves and a pump chamber which can be compressed through the skin to achieve drainage of ascitic fluid.[11]

In 1970, Summers described an implantable peristaltic pump for use in removing excess body fluid from the brain in hydrocephalus and from the peritoneal cavity in ascites. He also proposed that it could be attached to a flexible refillable fluid bladder and used as an infusion pump. An unusual feature of this device is that the implanted portion contains no power source and is driven through a magnetic coupling with an external drive unit. The device was used investigationally in several hydrocephalic infants.[12]

The Infuse-A-Port, developed by the Infusaid Corporation, is designed to provide prolonged access to a vein, artery, or body cavity for the administration of anticancer agents, blood, antibiotics, and other parenteral solutions. It consists of a self-sealing septum, a housing, and a cannula. Fluids to be administered can be injected or infused, using an extracorporeal pump, through the refill septum and from there into the desired location via the cannula.[13]

ACTIVE IMPLANTABLE INFUSION DEVICES

The primary focus of this chapter is on active implantable drug infusion devices designed for clinical use. Such a device contains an intrinsic power source that permits long-term in vivo operation. It also has some means of replacement of the infusate so that its functional lifetime is not limited by the volume of drug that can be placed in the reservoir. Development of devices of this type began about 1970 and followed two paths. One route of development arose from the need for a safe, reliable, and effective means for delivering parenteral drugs to outpatients. A single vapor pressure powered system was the outcome of this conceptual approach. A second line of development came from attempts by the diabetes research community to develop an implantable artificial pancreas for the control of diabetes. This developmental concept included mimicry of the pancreatic beta cell through the use of electronically mediated feedback control. Implantable pump development along these two lines is described in detail in the sections that follow.

History of Implantable Infusion Pump Development

Vapor Pressure Powered Pump

Background

In contrast to external prostheses such as artificial limbs, which date back many years, the development of totally implantable artificial organs is a comparatively recent phenomenon. Implantable artificial joints and implantable capsules for slow drug release were introduced in the 1930s, the artificial heart valve and the cardiac pacemaker in the 1950s, and the implantable infusion pump in the 1960s.

Conception and Initial Development

The first implantable pump developed to the stage of a commercially available medical product in widespread clinical use was conceived in August 1969 at the University of Minnesota Minneapolis, by Perry J. Blackshear, Frank D. Dorman, Perry L. Blackshear Jr., Richard L. Varco, and Henry Buchwald. I is a dual-chambered, disk-shaped device with an inexhaustable volatile liquid power source.[14] A stainless steel prototype wa built for bench testing in September 1969, and the first anima trials, initiated in January 1970, demonstrated that the devic could maintain heparin anticoagulation in dogs for severa days.[15] The University of Minnesota licensed the patent for this device to the Metal Bellows Corporation (Sharon, Mass.) in April 1971 for commercial development. After several design changes, the basic configuration that is in use today was developed in 1972. When initial in vivo studies demonstrated the viability of the new design, preclinical heparin infusion studies were initiated in June 1973. After 25 dogs had been successfully anticoagulated with heparin from implanted pumps for more than 6 months and a cohort of these for more than 1 year,[16] clinical studies were initiated.

Heparin Infusion in Ambulatory Subjects

The first human implantation of this device for any purpose was performed on Oct. 22, 1975 by Buchwald and colleagues for continuous heparin infusion in the treatment of recurrent venous thromboembolism.[17, 18] Further episodes of venous thromboembolism were prevented in these patients, most of whom were refractory to oral anticoagulant therapy.[19] Chapleau and Robertson introduced continuous heparin therapy by implantable infusion pump for the treatment of spontaneous high cervical carotid artery dissection.[20] After cerebral arteriography revealed a high-grade stenotic lesion of the distal left internal cervical carotid artery in a patient who had experienced a transient ischemic attack, an Infusaid pump was implanted on Aug. 16, 1979. After 5 months of continuous heparin infusion, repeat transfemoral cerebral arteriography revealed a normal left internal carotid artery and normal intracranial vessels. At that time, the reseachers concluded that continuous heparin therapy had been successful and was no longer necessary; the pump was removed.

Continuous Organ-Specific Cancer Chemotherapy

In January 1975, prior to the initiation of the first clinical trial with heparin, studies were begun at Minnesota in laboratory animals to assess the feasibility of using the pump for 5-FUDR infusion into the hepatic artery. One pump used in these studies was equipped with an auxiliary side port intended for use in arteriography to ascertain the infusion pattern of a drug on a regular basis. This feature was not included on pumps used in the first clinical trial with 5-FUDR because the bore of the catheter was too small to accommodate sufficient quantities of the highly viscous radiopaque contrast medium used for arteriography. The first series of human implantations of an implantable pump for cancer chemotherapy was initiated on June 7, 1977 by Buchwald et al.[21] This series, which included four subjects with secondary or primary nonresectable liver tumors who received continuous intra-arterial infusions of 5-FUDR from the implanted pumps, demonstrated the feasibility of organ-specific cancer chemotherapy using a totally implantable infusion system. Subsequently the Metal Bellows Corporation redesigned the auxiliary side injection port, in collaboration with Cohen et al.[22] and Ensminger et al.[23] for use in both liver scans and injection of additional cancer chemotherapeutic agents for adjuvant therapy. Suspensions of ^{99}Tc-macroaggregated albumin were injected through the side ports of implanted pumps by Cohen et al. and Ensminger et al. to perform low-flow radionuclide angiography at intervals throughout the course of therapy in their patients. In 1977 the Infusaid Corporation (Norwood, Mass.) was formed as a subsidiary of Metal Bellows Corporation specifically for implantable pump research and development and, in the future, for manufacturing and marketing. Thereafter, the pump model without the side port became known as the Infusaid Model 100 pump and that with the side port became known as the Infusaid Model 400 pump.

Intrathecal Morphine Infusion

The treatment of chronic intractable pain by the continuous intrathecal infusion of morphine from an Infusaid pump was pioneered by Onofrio et al.[24] They found that this treatment method maintained a pain-free state while preserving alertness and motor and sensory functions.

Continuous Insulin Infusion

When the Minnesota group began to consider the use of implantable pump technology in the treatment of diabetes, we initially viewed our device as the reservoir and pumping component of a totally artificial pancreas. Slow development of the implantable glucose sensor, in addition to our early successful experience with continuous insulin infusion, led us to conclude that continuous insulin infusion without feedback control might serve as a therapeutic alternative to conventional insulin therapy in insulin-requiring diabetics. Previous glucose tolerance studies in laboratory animals indicated that near-normal glucose responses to an IV glucose challenge could be maintained using a continuous single-rate insulin infusion pump.[25]

During insulin infusion experiments in laboratory animals, which began about 1977, we became acutely aware of the tendency of insulin solutions to clog the capillary flow restrictor of the pump (in contrast to heparin and 5-FUDR). Insulin precipitated and occluded nine pumps implanted in dogs within 43 days. Attempts to overcome this difficulty included modifications of both the pump and the infusate. Teflon capillary was substituted for stainless steel as the pump's flow restrictor to overcome a potential galvanic corrosion problem at the pump-flow restrictor junction to prevent local pH shifts that could precipitate insulin. A variety of combinations of insulin, buffers, and chelating agents were also tested for their ability to resist insulin precipitation. These included both zinc and zinc-free insulin, buffers (0.20M and 0.2M sodium acetate, 0.01M sodium phosphate, and glycine), and a chelating agent, ethylenediaminetetraacetic acid (EDTA). No combination prevented the precipitation of insulin in implantable pumps; plugging occurred despite maintenance of the pH of the insulin preparation in the pump within the soluble range.[26] Success in preventing insulin precipitation was finally achieved by the addition of 80% glycerol (v/v) to the infusate preparation. Glycerol is commonly added to peptide solutions to convey thermal stability. When implantable pump infusion studies in dogs, with glycerol added to the insulin infusate, demonstrated continued patency for more than 250 days each, we decided to initiate clinical trials of continuous insulin infusion in man.[27] These began on Oct. 25, 1980 with the implantation of the first Infusaid pump for insulin infusion.[28] In five patients with type II diabetes who were treated in this manner, the pump improved control of glycemia, as manifested by a reduction in mean plasma glucose, fasting glucose, and postprandial glucose levels, together with a diminution of glycemic excursions and normalization of glycosylated hemoglobin.[29] These individuals have now been studied for more than 2 years, with excellent patient acceptance of the device and without mishaps.

Conclusion

To date the Infusaid pump has been approved by the FDA for the delivery of heparin, 5-FUDR, and morphine. Approximately 10,000 Infusaid pumps have been implanted, most of them for cancer chemotherapy.

ELECTRICALLY POWERED PUMPS

The Artificial Pancreas Concept

During the 1960s, beginning attempts were made to develop an artificial endocrine pancreas that could respond to changes in plasma glucose levels with the administration of appropriate quantities of insulin or an insulin antagonist such as glucagon or glucose. Proponents of this concept hoped, in this way, to maintain normoglycemia in diabetic subjects using a negative feedback control system analogous to that utilized by the natural pancreas. Pioneering work on the development of an artificial device for the control of glycemia was reported by Kadish in 1964, who used a Technicon Autoanalyzer to analyze glucose concentrations in blood drawn through a double-lumen catheter at 0.2μl/hour.[30] By means of electronically controlled servomechanisms and a syringe pump, the device was designed to administer insulin if blood glucose exceeded 150 mg/dl or glucagon if it fell below 50 ml/dl. In a trial with a diabetic volunteer, the device responded to hypoglycemic and hyperglycemic challenges by returning blood glucose to the 50–150 mg/dl range, but its sluggish response time (10–11 minutes) allowed substantial glycemic excursions to occur. A further negative aspect of the device was that it used excessive amounts of blood (288 ml/day).

Pfeiffer et al.[31] and Albisser et al.[32] reported in 1974 that they were able to essentially normalize plasma glucose concentrations in diabetic volunteers. They used equipment similar to that used by Kadish but with several modifications. An improved version of the Technicon Autoanalyzer was used that reduced response time to 4–5 minutes and reduced blood loss per day of continuous operation to about 70 ml. They also developed control algorithms that altered insulin and insulin antagonist infusion rates according to rates of change in glycemic parameters as well as static plasma glucose values. These algorithms permitted the machines to anticipate glycemic excursions and respond accordingly. All of the devices described above were large extracorporeal units suitable only for acute studies in the hospital setting.

The Electrochemical Sensor

During the early 1970s, Soeldner of the Joslin Clinic and Bessman of University of Southern California (Los Angeles) began work on a miniaturized and simplified form of an artificial pancreas—more appropriately called an artificial beta cell—designed for implantation. As envisioned by Soeldner et al., such a device would consist of a glucose sensor with an accompanying power supply, a computer, a pump, and an insulin reservoir with a self-sealing refill portal.[33] They suggested that it could include such additional features as telemetered alarm signals to indicate device malfunction or the need to refill the reservoir. Based on the belief that the glucose sensor was the most important component of the system, they began that phase of development first.

In the Technicon Autoanalyzer—the equipment used by Albisser and Pfeiffer and colleagues for continuous plasma glucose determination—a continuous stream of blood is drawn from a patient through a double-lumen catheter, diluted, anticoagulated, and then dialyzed against alkaline potassium ferricyanide. The glucose level is then determined colorimetrically. While this method is satisfactory for the extracorporeal units described above, it is too cumbersome for an implantable system. Soeldner and colleagues chose instead to design an electrochemical sensor based on the property of nobel metals such as platinum to catalyze the oxidation of glucose to gluconic acid. Several electrochemical sensor subtypes can be constructed using this basic principle, including fuel cell, polarographic, potentiometric, and potentiodynamic systems. In 1973, Chang et al. of Soeldner's group chose the fuel cell type of sensor for their initial experiments.[34] A fuel cell is comprised of a nonconsumable catalytic anode and cathode, an electrolyte, and membranes separating the anodic and cathodic environments. The system does not need applied current or a reference electrode, thus reducing the problem of oxide formation and overcoming the problem of reference electrode degradation. Oxide coating on the platinum anode is reduced but not eliminated by the lack of applied current. The performance of eight of these sensors was tested by subcutaneous implantation in monkeys for up to 117 days. Sensor output, which was transmitted through percutaneous lead wires to an amplifier and recorder, was not strictly comparable with blood glucose values obtained by standard methods. However, sensor-derived values following meals and during glucose tolerance tests appeared to be within expected ranges.

One shortcoming of the electrochemical sensor is its nonspecificity. In addition to glucose, it responds to other monosaccharides, certain amino acids, ethanol, and urea. Since these substances are commonly found in blood and intracellular fluid, their presence can profoundly alter the accuracy of the results obtained by this method.

The Enzyme Electrode Sensor

Like Soeldner, Bessman and his colleagues chose the glucose sensor as the first component of their system for development. However, the type of unit they chose for development was an enzyme electrode sensor. Like the electrochemical sensor described above, the enzyme electrode catalyzes the oxidation of glucose to gluconic acid and hydrogen peroxide; unlike the electrochemical sensor, the enzyme electrode is highly specific for gluocose. The enzyme electrode glucose sensor, originally developed by Clark and Lyons about 1962,[35] consisted of a glucose oxidase solution sandwiched between semipermeable polymeric membranes. Initially, a pH electrode measured glucose concentrations as a function of hydrogen ion concentration, which changed in accordance with the amount of gluconic acid formed. Later designs potentiometrically measured glucose concentration as a function of oxygen depletion using an oxygen electrode, also designed by Clark.[36] In a modified enzyme electrode glucose sensor designed by Updike and Hicks, glucose oxidase was bound to a thin layer of polyacrylamide gel.[37] This sensor substantially reduced response times over previous sensor models. It differed from the previous model of Clark by using a polarographic rather than a potentiometric oxygen electrode, i.e., it measured amperage rather than voltage differences.

Bessman and Schultz modified the Clark design further by immobilizing and stabilizing the glucose oxidase by intramolecular and intermolecular cross-linkages in cloth matrix disks that were cemented over the plastic membrane of a polarographic oxygen electrode.[38] This modification, reported in 1973, extended the useful range of the device up to 400 mg/dl, about twice that of the Updike-Hicks sensor. The pumping system designed by Thomas and Bessman to accompany the glucose sensor consisted of two opposed piezoelectric disk benders, arranged in opposition to form a bellows, connected to a solenoid valve.[39] A rectangular wave pulse generator activates the opening and closing of the solenoid valve and, through a step-up transformer, activates the flexing of the disk benders. The system was capable of delivering insulin in pulses of 0.2 μl or less; delivery rate in this device is a function of the number of pulses per unit time. Prior to 1977, Bessman et al. implanted a pump of this design in an alloxan diabetic dog with insulin delivered into the peritoneal cavity.[40] They reported that plasma glucose was maintained within the physiologic range for 4 days using this system.

Is Glucose Sensing Necessary?

Although the implantable glucose sensor was originally considered to be the most essential component in the artificial β cell idea, its development was hindered by a variety of technical problems, including the tendency of the body to encapsulate it and disrupt communication with the surrounding serum or intracellular fluid. Therefore, some investigators began to explore the concept that devices without feedback control might be suitable for restoring normoglycemia in many subjects with diabetes. Slama et al. conducted the first study of this type.[41] They administered continuous IV infusions of insulin to seven diabetic volunteers using portable peristaltic pumps. At mealtimes, the insulin solution used for basal insulin delivery was replaced with one 15 times more concentrated. Very good control of glycemia was achieved in this study, but it was not significantly better than what they were able to achieve using a regimen of multiple insulin injections. This study demonstrated the feasibility of controlling glycemia using continuous insulin infusion without feedback control, but it also showed the difficulty of maintaining long-term vascular access for drug infusion with a portable device. Infusion of insulin had to be prematurely discontinued in three patients because of inflammation at the cannulation site.

After Slama's study was reported in 1974, several other investigators performed similar studies using portable pumps, with gradually improving success. Pickup and colleagues demonstrated that insulin infused subcutaneously through a small needle can maintain excellent glucoregulation and, for the most part, alleviate the problem of vascular access, since the infusion site can easily be moved to a new location if the existing one becomes inflamed.[42] Tamborlane and associates demonstrated that plasma glucose levels could be normalized in brittle juvenile diabetics using techniques similar to those described by Pickup et al.[43] These studies indicated that automatic feedback control is not essential to achieve excellent control. In the above cases, feedback was provided by the physicians and patients, who used data from multiple daily capillary blood glucose determinations to adjust insulin delivery rates.

Implantable Systems Without Feedback Control

In 1975, Shumakov (USSR) described an implantable, inductively recharged, electronically controlled insulin infusion system with a percutaneously refillable reservoir and a micrometering pump that administered microdoses of insulin every 5 minutes as a basal infusion rate. By using a control unit about the size of a cigarette pack, the device could be commanded to deliver additional mealtime doses of insulin. The mode of operation of the device could be changed by external command. Animal and clinical experience was mentioned but no results were given or subsequently published.[44]

One of the major proponents of the electronically controlled implantable infusion pump in the United States was William Spencer, then of Sandia Laboratories, who began by designing several investigational extracorporeal insulin infusion pumps,[45, 46] and later, in collaboration with Eaton and Schade of the University of New Mexico (Albuquerque), developed the first successful implantable programmable insulin pump. Spencer's presentation at the Workshop on Artificial Devices for the Control of Blood Glucose, held in Bethesda, Maryland on December 1–2, 1977, was probably a major impetus for the subsequent surge in interest in programmable implantable drug infusion pumps that occurred throughout the medical device industry.[46] At this meeting, he presented the concept of an inductively programmable electronic beta cell in which feedback control was supplied by the physician or patient. Interest was also stimulated by the awarding of several contracts for insulin pump development by the National Institute of Arthritis, Metabolism and Digestive Disease. Subsequently, the implantable, rotary solenoid-driven, peristaltic pump, developed jointly by Sandia Laboratories and the University of New Mexico, was successfully tested in infusion studies in diabetic dogs[47] and then implanted in a type I diabetic human subject by Schade, Eaton, and colleagues on Jan. 7, 1981.[48]

In Europe, Siemens AG (Erlangen, Federal Republic of Germany) developed and evaluated programmable bedside syringe pumps[49] and portable peristaltic pumps[50–52] before initiating clinical studies using an implantable unit of their design. A Siemens Model DFA 01 implantable programmable peristaltic pump was implanted in a human type I diabetic on April 8, 1981 by Irsigler and associates of the Boltzmann Institute for Metabolic Disease, Vienna.[53]

Conclusion

To date, the artificial pancreas concept has led to development to the stage of clinical trial of two programmable, implantable, peristaltic insulin pumps. These successful developments involved the collaborative efforts of university professors, government scientists, and representatives of private industry both in the United States and Europe.

Current Implantable Infusion Pump Technology

Three basic types of pumping mechanisms have been utilized in implantable infusion devices. They are (1) the vapor pressure powered pump, (2) the peristaltic pump, and (3) the pulsatile solenoid pump. Of these, the vapor pressure powered pump is FDA approved and has been the subject of substantial clinical study. The peristaltic pumping mechanism appears to be the most popular approach but, at the present time, has had only limited clinical exposure. The pulsatile solenoid pump mechanism is being investigated in animal studies but has not been introduced into the clinical setting. These three basic types of pumps are reviewed from an engineering standpoint in the first part of this section. In the second part, some novel pump designs that use alternative modes of delivery will be reviewed; none of these has as yet advanced to the stage of being a serious contender in the clinical armamentarium. The third part reviews some of the characteristics an infusate must have to be suitable for use in an implantable pump.

ENGINEERING ASPECTS OF THREE IMPLANTABLE PUMP TYPES

Vapor Pressure Powered Pump

At present, the only vapor pressure powered pump available is that invented at the University of Minnesota[14, 15] and manufactured by the Infusaid Corporation. Its principle of operation is the basic physicochemical concept that at a given temperature, a liquid in equilibrium with its vapor phase exerts a constant pressure which is independent of enclosing volume. Design criteria for this infusion system were that it must be constructed of biocompatible materials, refillable by percutaneous injection, small enough to avoid encumbering the recipient but with a large enough reservoir to permit a long interval between refills, and rechargeable without surgical intervention. In accordance with these criteria, a disk-shaped, titanium, two-chambered pump was developed in which a volatile charging fluid in equilibrium with its vapor phase is sealed in the outer chamber. The charging fluid is selected to provide an appropriate vapor pressure at physiologic temperatures. The drug to be infused is placed in the inner chamber, which is accessible by means of a self-sealing septum. The two chambers are separated by a flexible metal bellows. Vapor pressure from the charging fluid compresses the bellows and expels the infusate through a bacterial filter, a capillary flow restrictor, and an infusion cannula into the desired body site. When the reservoir of the pump is refilled by percutaneous needle injection through the refill septum, the expansion of the bellows compresses and condenses the charging fluid vapor and recharges the pump. Thus, the pump is refilled and recharged simultaneously.

The flow rate of the pump is determined by the length and internal diameter of the capillary flow restrictor through which the infusate must pass as it exits the pump. Flow through such a tube is governed by the Poisseuille equation:

$$Q = \frac{\pi D^4 \, \Delta P}{120 \, \mu l}$$

where Q is the flow rate, D is the internal diameter of the capillary tube, δP is the change in viscosity across the capillary tube, μ is the viscosity of the infusate, and l is the length of the capillary tube.

Thus, when δP, D and l are fixed, as is the case once a pump is manufactured, the only means of changing the flow rate in situ is to alter the viscosity of the infusate. Drug delivery rate can, of course, be adjusted by changing the concentration of drug in the infusate. An external view of the Infusaid pump is shown in Figure 1. The Model 100 device is 72 mm in diameter by 25 mm in height and weighs 180 gm.

The vapor pressure powered pump has the advantages of an indefinitely long in vivo lifetime and the potential for high volumetric efficiency. One concern often expressed by physicians introduced to the device is its sensitivity to changes in ambient temperature and pressure. The infusate delivery rate is proportional to the difference (δP) between the reservoir pressure of the pump and that at its cannula tip. δP is increased when the vapor pressure of the charging fluid increases (e.g., during febrile states) and when the pressure at the catheter tip decreases (e.g., when altitude increases); venous pressure differs by only a few millimeters of water from atmospheric pressure. Both a 1° F change in temperature and a 1,000-ft change in altitude cause an approximate 6% change in the pump's flow rate. Flow rate variation due to changes in ambient temperature and pressure, of sufficient magnitude to warrant intervention, has occurred only once in our 8 years' clinical experience. In that case, we elected to administer protamine sulfate to a

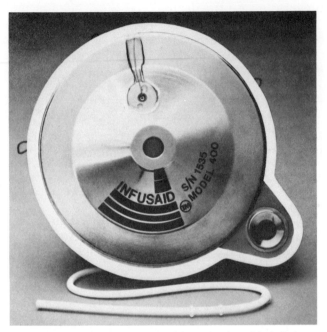

Fig 1.—External view of the Infusaid Model 400 implantable infusion pump developed jointly by University of Minnesota and Infusaid Corporation. (Photo courtesy of Infusaid Corporation.)

patient who was receiving heparin from the pump and whose coagulation times became abnormally elevated when she became febrile during a bout of pneumonia. Her fever was controlled with antipyretics within 24 hours and protamine was discontinued. Although flow rate variation due to temperature and pressure changes has not caused significant difficulty in our patients, most of whom live on the relatively level terrain of the midwestern United States, the management of subjects who change altitude frequently, such as airline pilots and mountain dwellers, could be troublesome. For this reason, we designed an infusion regulator that compensates for ambient temperature and pressure variability.[54]

The infusion regulator consists of a titanium diaphragm suspended above an O ring metering port. Differences between pump and cannula pressures deflect the diaphragm so that the metering port opens when the pressure decreases and closes when the pressure increases. Thus, the pressure difference across the capillary flow restrictor and therefore the flow rate remain constant by feedback control, as long as the viscosity of the infusate remains unchanged. The set point pressure difference of this component is determined by diaphragm thickness, modulus of elasticity, and the distance the diaphragm must deflect to close the metering port. In performance tests of a pump equipped with an infusion regulator, flow rate changed 0.3% per 1° F change in temperature and 0.6% per 1,000-ft change in elevation, in contrast to the 6% changes under these same conditions in unregulated pumps.[54]

It is feasible to modify the Infusaid pump to provide more than one flow rate without sacrificing the advantages gained by its inexhaustible power source. This can be accomplished by dividing the capillary flow restrictor into two segments connected by a transcutaneously magnetically manipulated valve. This action increases flow rate in proportion to the ratio of the lengths of the two segments. Either a latching or a nonlatching valve can be used. Pumps of this type have been used successfully in a number of laboratory studies of insulin infusion in diabetic dogs.[55-57] Pump models have also been developed for experimental use that have an arrangement of two valves that cannot be opened simultaneously and an accumulator that holds a prandial dose. One valve fills the accumulator; the other allows the accumulator to empty over a preselected time interval.

Peristaltic Pump

At present, the most popular design for an implantable programmable drug delivery system uses a peristaltic pumping mechanism, battery power, and electronic controls. Briefly, a peristaltic pump consists of a flexible tube placed in a U-shaped chamber in contact with rollers that press against the tube with sufficient force to occlude its lumen. The rollers are mounted on a rotor and rotated by a motor. As the rollers move and compress the lumen of the tube, fluid is moved toward the exit. The rollers and housing are arranged so that a second roller begins to squeeze the tube before the first disengages. This prevents backflow of the infusate. The peristaltic mechanism is one commonly used in the past for drug infusion from portable pumps. For example, the Watkins Chronofuser, a spring-driven portable pump developed in the early 1960s for the administration of cancer chemotherapeutic agents, is so designed.[58]

Currently, at least three groups have developed implantable pumps with peristaltic pumping mechanisms. They are Sandia Laboratories, Siemens AG, and Medtronic Inc. Of these, the pump developed by Sandia Laboratories is most thoroughly described in the literature.

SANDIA PUMP.—In the Sandia system a three-roller peristaltic pump head is driven by a rotary solenoid motor. The electromagnetic components of the system are made of an iron-cobalt alloy; most of the remaining components are made of stainless steel. The rotary solenoid driver is a type of stepper motor which rotates in uniform steps. However, it generates more torque than a conventional stepper motor of the same volume because every pole on the solenoid rotor is attracted to its corresponding stator pole. The pump head is designed so that each roller gradually decompresses the tube from fully closed to fully open over a 120° rotation. With the three-roller head, at least one roller completely occludes the tube at all times.

Implanted electronic microcircuitry controls pump function and stores for patient or physician access flow rate, battery status, and other diagnostic information regarding the unit. The control unit consists of 26 complementary metal oxide semiconductor (CMOS) components enclosed in eight leadless, hermetically sealed packages, with a 32-kHz watch crystal for timing. A parylene coating was added to protect against moisture. Power is provided by two hermetically sealed 3.66-V lithium-thionyl chloride AA batteries connected in series.

Two-way communication between the implanted pump and an external hand-held programmer is achieved by inductive coupling with a 30-kHz carrier frequency. The programmer contains an RCA 1802D CMOS microprocessor with 1024 bytes of read only memory (ROM) and 128 bytes of random access memory (RAM). Battery power is provided by two cells identical to those used in the implantable unit. A four-button keyboard is provided for patient or physician interaction with the programmer's output that can be read from a liquid crystal display.

The system provides 15 low flow rates and 15 high doses. Low infusion rates range from 0.39 to 5.9 units per hour; high doses range from 0.84 to 12.5 units of U-100 insulin. Insulin is delivered in uniform 21-μl pulses. The infusion rate is determined by the number of pulses per unit time.

The batteries, electronics, and inductive communication coil are hermetically sealed in one half of a titanium enclosure; the rotary solenoid pump is housed in the other half, with the two compartments separated by a header plate. Hermetic single electrode feedthroughs in the header plate are used to provide electrical connections between the battery and electronics with the pump. Titanium tubing feedthroughs in the wall of the pump enclosure permit entry of the silicone rubber tube from the reservoir and exit of the delivery catheter. The insulin reservoir is a disk-shaped silicone rubber pouch with a hard plastic (polystyrene) needle stop and septum housing. It has a 5-ml capacity and is designed to be implanted as a separate unit, connected to but separate from the pump module. The reservoir is connected to the pump module using silicone rubber tubing of dimensions 0.7 mm inside diameter (ID) $\times$ 2.4 mm outside diameter (OD); the peristaltic pump tubing is 1.5 mm ID $\times$ 3.0 mm OD; and the drug delivery catheter is a modified silicone rubber cerebrospinal fluid peritoneal catheter with a low-pressure slit valve at the distal end.[59]

In vitro and in vivo preclinical testing revealed both limiting and useful features of the present design. Because of the permeability of silicone rubber tubing to water vapor, the rotary solenoid pump was exposed to 100% relative humidity during operation. Considerable corrosion and pitting was noted in rotor and stator parts that were not coated with nickel in units evaluated in bench tests. More extensive nickel plating of motor components was planned for future studies. The silicone rubber peristaltic pump tubing became slightly distorted and developed microscopic cracks on the inside surface; no adverse effects due to these changes were noted. A steady decline in battery output occurred over time due to the development of a passivation layer of lithium chloride on the lithium electrode of the cell. Because of this phenomenon, predicted battery lifetimes of 31 months were not realized and functional durations of 6 months were common. A capacitor discharge system is expected to substantially lengthen battery performance time. Perhaps the weakest component of the system is the separate silicone rubber reservoir module, which is highly vulnerable to damage.[59] Indeed, a reservoir leak occurred during initial clinical studies with this device.[48]

On the positive side, pump performance in clinical trials was successful, with normalization of glycosylated hemoglobin in addition to mean plasma glucose.[48] Remote programming of drug infusion rates and interrogation of pump status worked well.[59] The device is shown in Figure 2.

The implantable pump technology developed by Sandia Laboratories has now been transferred to Shiley Incorporated (Irvine, Calif.) for the development of commercially suitable pump designs.

SIEMENS PUMP.—A peristaltic pumping mechanism is also used in the Promedos ID1, the implantable pump developed by Siemens AG. Like the Sandia device, the Siemens device is driven by a stepper motor electronically controlled by means of a hand-held programmer. In addition to the peristaltic pump and stepper motor, components of the implantable unit include a battery, control electronics, and a 10-ml drug reservoir that can be refilled by percutaneous needle injection through a self-sealing septum. Unlike the Sandia pump, the reservoir in the Promedos ID1 is sealed with the pump's titanium capsule. The

Fig 2.—The implantable, rotary solenoid-driven pump developed by Sandia Laboratories and University of New Mexico. (Photo courtesy of J.E. Love, Sandia Laboratories.)

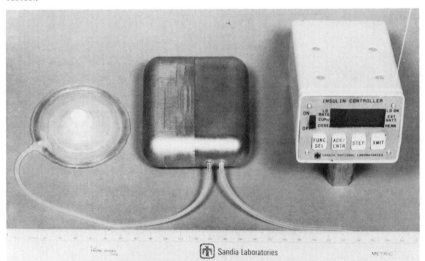

interior of the capsule is maintained at negative pressure to prevent fluid loss into the body in the event of a leak. The pump can provide 12 different basal rates, from 1 to 15 µl/hour, and 12 higher rates that can be superimposed on each basal rate on demand. The demand rate is switched off automatically after 1 hour.[60, 61] To date no clinical study results have been reported using the Promedos ID1 pump. Previous reports of clinical studies using Siemens pumps published by Irsigler and colleagues[53] and Selam and associates[62, 63] used an earlier pump model, the Siemens DFA 01. Dimensions of the Promedose ID1 are 85 × 60 × 22 mm. Its weight is 170 gm. An external view of the device is shown in Figure 3.

MEDTRONIC PUMP.—Like the Sandia and Siemens devices, the Medtronic pump (models 8600, 8601) utilizes a peristaltic pump driven by a stepper motor to deliver infusate. The device is powered by a lithium thionyl chloride battery with an estimated functional lifetime of 2 years and is controlled by microprocessor-based hybrid electronics. Infusate is stored in a flexible 20-ml titanium reservoir. Programming options include

Fig 3.—The Siemens Promedose 1 implantable dosing device. (Photo courtesy of Siemens AG.)

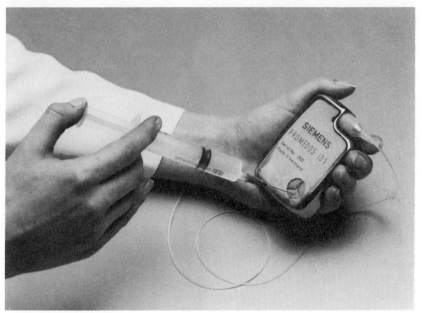

intermittent doses, continuous infusion, and boluses of a variety of waveforms. Programming is performed telemetrically using a portable desktop computer with "user friendly" software. The unit is 70 mm in diameter by 27 mm in height and weighs 175 gm.[60, 61, 64, 65] It is shown in Figure 4. To date, Medtronic pumps have been implanted in 27 patients for the administration of intrathecal morphine, intra-arterial 5-FUDR, and IV Adriamycin.[65]

Fig 4.—The Medtronic implantable pump. (Photo courtesy of Medtronic Inc.)

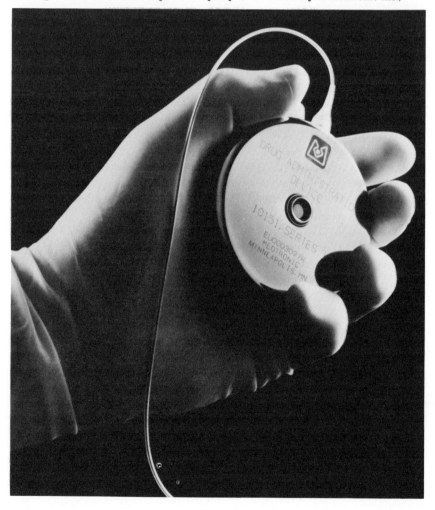

Pulsatile Solenoid Pump

An alternative approach to fluid delivery of an infusate from a programmable implantable pump was taken by Fischell and colleagues at the Johns Hopkins University Applied Physics Laboratory. Their implantable device—called the Implantable Programmable Infusion Pump (IPIP)—uses a solenoid-driven reciprocating chamber with attendant check valves to move infusate from the reservoir out through the delivery catheter. This pulsatile pump delivers infusate in pulses of 2 µl, utilizing less than 2 µW power for each. Infusate is stored in a 7.2-ml flexible diaphragm reservoir maintained at a pressure of 4 psi to preclude loss of drugs into the subcutaneous tissues if a leak in the fluid path occurs. The reservoir is filled through a refill septum located at the bottom of a ceramic cone. The unit is powered by a lithium thionyl chloride battery calculated to provide more than 10 years of in vivo function. A system of CMOS microelectronics with a microprocessor and 8 kilobytes of RAM controls the device. It can provide any of eight different insulin infusion waveforms in response to external commands. The system is designed so that programming and interrogation of the unit can be accomplished using appropriate ancillary equipment linked via telephone. An assembled IPIP, manufactured by Pacesetter Systems, Sylmar, Calif. is shown in Figure 5. Externally the IPIP is 81 mm in diameter and 20 mm thick; its weight is 170 gm.[60, 61, 66, 67] The device is currently being tested in laboratory animals.

OTHER PUMP DESIGNS

At present, three basic pump designs are at some stage of commercial development. As described above, the vapor pressure powered pump developed at the University of Minnesota is being manufactured by the Infusaid Corporation. Three peristaltic pump designs are being developed by Siemens AG, Medtronic Inc., and Shiley Inc., the latter developed originally by Sandia Laboratories. A pulsatile solenoid pump design devised by workers at Johns Hopkins University has been licensed to Pacesetter Systems for commercial development.

Two pump types that have been evaluated in laboratory

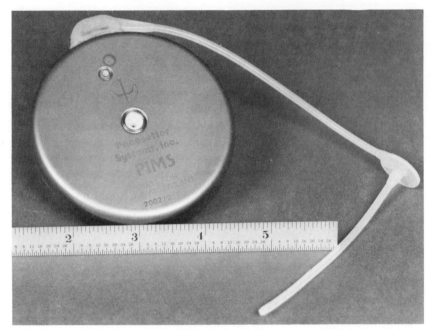

Fig 5.—The Implantable Programmable Infusion Pump developed by Johns Hopkins University and Pacesetters, Inc. (Photo courtesy of R.E. Fischell, Johns Hopkins University.)

studies but have not reached the stage of commercial development are the piezoelectric and foam transport designs.

Piezoelectric Design

The use of flexing piezoelectric disk benders as a means of pumping infusate from an implantable pump was described by Thomas and Bessman[39] as a component of their artificial beta cell. This type of system is based on the property of piezoceramic material to increase or decrease in size when positive or negative voltages are applied. In a piezoelectric pump, thin piezoceramic disks are bonded to the flexible metal ends of a short cylindrical chamber. As the disks contract or expand in response to the applied voltage, the ends of the chamber bulge in and out, with a resultant pumping effect. Unidirectional fluid flow is achieved by the addition of electrically activated valves in appropriate phase with the electrical impulses sent to the disks. The voltages required to achieve an adequate piezoceramic flexing effect are very small; thus, this type of pumping system is potentially very attractive for an implantable pump when available power is limited. However, energy-efficient valves are also needed if the resultant system is to be applicable for implantable use. In the system described by Bessman and colleagues the miniature solenoid valve consumed two thirds of the power available for the entire system.[68] Spencer et al. described a system similar to that of Bessman and associates that substituted piezoelectric valves for the solenoid valve in order to reduce power consumption.[45] A modification of the vapor pressure powered pump that uses a piezoelectric pumping valve as an infusate metering device was described by Schubert et al.[69] Piezoelectric pumps with glucose sensors designed by Bessman et al. were implanted in seven dogs for evaluation.[68] These studies were limited to a few days each because of the relatively high power consumption of the implantable units.

Foam Transport Design

A novel pump design for insulin administration was introduced by Sefton et al.[70] Basal delivery is provided by transport of infusate through a hydrophilic polyurethane foam; augmented delivery is accomplished by activating a solenoid-driven piston that repeatedly squeezes the foam to release the drug at a higher rate. The device contains only one moving part and requires no valves. The device is currently being tested in pancreatectomized dogs.[71]

INFUSATE CONSIDERATIONS

To be suitable for use in implantable pumps, an infusate must be stable at physiologic temperatures, compatible with standard pump materials, and available in concentrations sufficient to allow a reasonable interval between refills. These criteria are met by heparin, 5-FUDR, and morphine, the first drugs approved by the FDA for clinical administration by implantable pump. However, 5-fluorouracil, an antitumor agent less expensive than and more widely used than 5-FUDR, is available only in concentrations so low that pump refilling would be required every 1–2 days to achieve therapeutic drug levels.

An unexpected problem arose when attempts were made to use insulin as an infusate. Investigators found that insulin tended to form aggregates or insoluble precipitates that clogged flow passages of implantable pumps, necessitating pump removal. A National Conference on Diabetes sponsored by the National Institutes of Health in 1979 concluded that "almost all investigators agreed that a major (perhaps the major) impediment to long-term continuous insulin delivery is the aggregation of insulin into crystals and sludge which blocks tubing, membranes, and pump. System failure almost always results. To date neither change in type or formulation of insulin nor change in system components has resolved this critical problem."[72] The aggregational behavior of insulin as it relates to infusion devices has been reviewed in detail elsewhere.[73, 74] Although advances have been made toward the development of an insulin preparation suitable for pump use, this goal remains elusive. Insulin preparations containing 80% glycerol have now been administered by Infusaid pumps in more than 100 patients for up to 2½ years without interruption of flow. A limitation of these preparations, however, is their tendency to form insulin oligomers with concomitant loss of bioactivity.[27] The *Insulin Delivery Workgroup Report* from the Second National Conference on Diabetes, held in Reston, Virginia, on Sept. 25–28, 1983, concluded that "further basic as well as applied research is needed to develop new insulins and their preparations suitable for use in external and implantable insulin delivery devices."[75]

Insulin is the first proteinaceous drug to be seriously investigated as a candidate for administration by implantable pump. That so much difficulty has been encountered in making insulin preparations compatible with infusion pumps may portend a challenging future in adapting peptide drug preparations for use in pumps. However, peptides will undoubtedly be a very important class of pump infusates, given their vulnerability to gastric acid and enzymes and because the new recombinant DNA technology promises to increase their availability at reduced costs. The benefits that can potentially be achieved by the ability to deliver these drugs to selected sites on a long-term basis will likely more than justify the effort expended to develop pump-compatible peptide infusates.

Clinical Application of Implantable Pump Technology

SURGICAL CONSIDERATIONS

Techniques for the surgical placement of the Infusaid, Siemens, and Sandia pumps have been described by a number of investigators. Surgical methods of implantation vary somewhat, based on the site of drug delivery, the configuration of the pump, and the preference of the surgeon. IV, intraperitoneal, intra-arterial, and intrathecal infusion sites have been used from pumps implanted subcutaneously or intramuscularly. Both abdominal and pectoral locations have been chosen for pump placement.

IV Infusion

One of the most common implantation sites for systemic drug delivery is a subcutaneous pocket in the subclavicular fossa with the delivery cannula placed for IV delivery. This site is often selected for the placement of cardiac pacemaker pulse generators. The pump's radiopaque cannula is threaded into the superior vena cava under direct fluoroscopic observation using a technique similar to that used for the insertion of cardiac pacemaker lead wires. The implantation procedure can be performed under local anesthesia. Surgical methods for the placement of a pump in the subclavicular fossa have been described in detail by Buchwald[76] and Hagmueller.[77] The techniques described are comparable. Both recommended cannulating the cephalic vein in the deltoid groove and threading the cannula into the superior vena cava via the axillary vein. Hagmueller proposed an additional alternative technique of splitting the fascia of the pectoral muscle beneath the clavicle just prior to the junction of the pectoral veins with the subclavian vein.

Placement of a drain in the pump pocket to avoid collection of serous fluid was originally recommended by both authors. At the University of Minnesota, we continue to place a drain to facilitate management of a pump site hematoma should it occur in the newly formed pump pocket following the initiation of heparin therapy. This usually necessitates that the patient remain hospitalized for 4–5 days until drainage stops and the Hemovac drain is removed. For applications other than heparin infusion, a pressure bandage is now placed over the pump and patients can usually return home 1 day postoperatively. With further refinements in technique, it is conceivable that in the future pump implantation may be done as an outpatient procedure.

Possibly due to relatively poor experience with percutaneous subclavian catheters for hyperalimentation and other purposes, it has been suggested that IV delivery by implanted pump carries a high risk for thrombosis.[78] We have now treated a total of 39 subjects with IV (superior vena cava) infusions of insulin for more than 458 patient-months. To date, no evidence of superior vena caval syndrome, pulmonary embolism, or other indications of catheter-associated thrombosis has been noted. In a previous (unpublished) study performed in our laboratory, a veterinary pathologist examined lung tissue from six dogs with implantable pumps in place from 1.5 to 30 months and found no evidence of microemboli. Additionally, postmortem gross and histologic examinations of the venal caval intima in contact with indwelling catheters from these pumps revealed no evidence of thromboembolic activity. This is consistent with the low incidence of severe thromboembolic complications associated with cardiac pacemaker implantation[79] and hyperalimentation lines.[80]

The IV route appears to facilitate the achievement of good metablic control in diabetes, to be easily accessible for implantation under local anesthesia, and to be relatively free of documented complications.[81] Thus, it is a prime candidate for the implantation site of choice for general drug delivery.

Intraperitoneal Infusion

Implantation of a pump for intraperitoneal insulin infusion has been described by Schade et al.[48] Irsigler et al.[53] Kritz et al.[81] and Selam et al.[62] The Sandia pump implanted by Schade et al. consisted of two implantable components, a titanium-encased pump and a silicone rubber reservoir, connected by a short segment of silicone rubber tubing. The pump was implanted in a submuscular site; the reservoir was placed in a subcutaneous location to make it accessible for refilling. The catheter was inserted into the peritoneal cavity by means of a 2-mm incision in the posterior rectus sheath and the parietal peritoneum. Surgical implantation was performed under general anesthesia. There were no difficulties with the implantation site per se, but the pump's silicone rubber reservoir had to be replaced after 2 weeks of infusion because it developed a leak.

Selam et al. utilized an intramuscular implantation site for the placement of a Siemens pump. Under general anesthesia, an 8-cm paraumbilical horizontal incision was made in the left lateral abdomen. The pump was implanted into the space between the internal oblique and the rectus and transversus muscles. The catheter was inserted into the peritoneal cavity through the linea alba. Swelling, lymphorrhea, and mild local discomfort to the patient developed 3 weeks after implantation. Lymphorrhea was eliminated after approximately 2 months, but mild discomfort and swelling persisted.

Irsigler et al., Kritz et al., and Hagmueller[77] described subcutaneous implantation of the Siemens and the Infusaid pumps for intraperitoneal infusion. Under local anesthesia, an 8–10-cm pararectal vertical skin incision was made in the left upper abdomen. The catheter was threaded through an opening made by blunt dissection of the rectus abdominis and fixed to the parietal peritoneum with two sutures. The pump was placed subcutaneously over the fascia of the external oblique abdominal muscle. Except for the development of adhesions in certain patients, no difficulties have been noted with this technique, which has now been used in approximately 60 subjects.

The intraperitoneal route offers the advantage of relatively easy catheter placement. The subcutaneous position of the pump appears to be preferable to intramuscular or submuscular sites because the operation can be performed under local anesthesia and seems to have fewer complications. Encapsulation of the catheter by peritoneal tissue and the formation of adhesions are potential problems that need further evaluation.

Intra-Arterial Infusion

In their first implantation of an implantable pump for cancer chemotherapy, Buchwald et al.[21] chose to follow the cannulation technique previously described by Watkins and Sullivan[82] for intrahepatic arterial infusion using the Chronometric Infuser. By this technique, under general anesthesia, the catheter was threaded into the hepatic artery via the gastroduodenal or gastroepiploic arteries at laparotomy. Correct positioning of the cannula was originally ascertained using fluorescein dye under direct observation using a Woods lamp. The body of the pump was placed in a subcutaneous pocket created in the abdominal wall by sharp dissection. Infusaid Model 100 pumps were used in these initial studies. For subsequent studies, a side port was added to the pump (Infusaid Model 400) and angiography has been performed directly through the side port using ^{99}Tc macroaggregated albumen[13] for confirming catheter position. It is essential to obtain a selective arteriogram of the hepatic and superior mesenteric arteries preoperatively to ascertain the origins of the patient's hepatic arterial blood supply.

Cohen et al.[83] described a transaxillary angiographic hepatic arterial catheterization technique. The implantation is performed under local anesthesia. Through a 2–3-cm incision in the shoulder, a polyethylene catheter is threaded into the hepatic artery under direct fluoroscopic vision. An Infusaid Model 400 pump is then implanted subcutaneously in the subclavicular fossa and its silicone rubber catheter connected to the polyethylene catheter by means of a friction connector. Among the 20 patients who have received intrahepatic arterial infusion of cancer chemotherapeutic agents by this technique, no arm vascular complications, hepatic arterial occlusions, peripheral emboli, pump malfunctions, or catheter occlusions occurred during 3,210 patient-days of operation. Three catheter migrations occurred in two patients; these required repositioning. Three cracked catheters required replacement.

Intraspinal Infusion

The first placement of an implantable pump for intrathecal morphine infusion was performed by Onofrio et al.[24] In this case, the pump (Infusaid Model 100) was implanted under local anesthesia in a pocket dissected beneath the right pectoralis major muscle. The catheter was tunneled beneath the serratus anterior and latissimus dorsi muscles and through the right paraspinous muscles into the spinal laminectomy wound. A partial bilateral hemilaminectomy was performed at T10 and T11 and the catheter was threaded intradurally to the T12 segment. The wounds were closed without drains.

A technique for pump implantation for epidural infusion was described by Harbaugh et al.[84] Briefly, under regional epidural anesthesia, the patient is positioned on his or her side. Catheter position is selected based on dermatologic levels involved in the patient's pain syndrome. Several vertebrae below the selected catheter site, a 5-cm vertical midline incision is made. A modified No. 9 Tuohy needle is placed in the epidural space. The silicone rubber catheter is passed over a cardiovascular guide wire and then directed under fluoroscopic control to the appropriate level of the epidural space. Water-soluble myelographic contrast medium is injected through the catheter to confirm that it is correctly placed. A subcutaneous pocket is then made on the anterior abdominal wall and the pump is placed within it. The epidural catheter is then tunneled subcutaneously to the pump site and connected to the pump's outlet catheter with a straight metal connector.

CLINICAL RESULTS TO DATE

Heparin

In most instances, with prompt and proper treatment, recurrences of thromboembolic disease can be prevented. However, for individuals whose disease does not respond to conventional oral modes of therapy, medical science heretofore had few good alternatives to offer. Therapeutic choices included prolonged hospitalization to receive heparin, vena caval ligation or umbrella placement, or inadequate oral drug or minidose heparin therapy, with the continuous risk of sudden death from pulmonary embolism. Obviously, the expense and life-style restrictions of prolonged hospitalization makes that an unsuitable alternative. Vena caval interruption generally causes poor drainage of the lower extremities with accompanying swelling, pain, and disability and may not prevent further pulmonary embolism, since collateral veins can become greatly enlarged and sometimes allow large thrombi to migrate to the lung. Warfarin and its derivatives and minidose heparin therapy (two to three daily subcutaneous injections of 5,000 units each) are effective in many patients but are ineffective in individuals with thromboembolic disease who are candidates for a pump. The Minnesota groups studied the effects of long-term heparin infusion by implantable pump in 21 patients with recurrent venous thromboembolism, most of whom failed conventional forms of therapy.[19] Continuous heparin infusion (mean delivery rate, 22,500 units/day) was maintained at 0.1–0.3 units/ml of plasma. Pumps were refilled by percutaneous needle injection every 4–8 weeks. Marked reduction of pain and improvement of mobility were reported by several patients with vena caval ligature syndrome. Recurrences of thromboembolic events were prevented by this regimen in all except one patient, who apparently was refractory to heparin as well as oral anticoagulant therapy. There were no spontaneous hemorrhagic episodes, but pump site hematomas occurred in several instances as a result of heparin spillage during pump refills. The refill technique has since been modified to eliminate this difficulty. Bone mineral densities of patients that had been receiving heparin for 1 year (1.00 ± 0.06 (SE) gm/cm) were not significantly different from baseline values (0.98 ± 0.08), but osteoporosis did occur in one subject.[19] In a subsequent study of longer mean duration (2 years), a 24% incidence of heparin-associated osteoporosis was noted.

While the population of individuals with refractory venous thromboembolism is small, it constitutes a group whose needs were not being met by conventional medical techniques. In some cases, heparin infusion by pump has led to dramatic improvements in mobility and freedom from pain with concomitant improvements in life-style. The Infusaid pump has been approved by the FDA for chronic heparin administration. Its use in the treatment of chronic thromboembolic disease, uncontrolled by other methods, has been designated an established procedure by Blue Cross and Blue Shield.[78] Chapleau and Robertson at the University of Tennessee are investigating the utility of this form of therapy in the treatment of patients who present with transient ischemic attacks uncorrectable by surgery.

Cancer Chemotherapy

Clinical experience to date using implantable pumps in the treatment of cancer has been reviewed recently by Chute and Buchwald.[85] Therefore our comments will be brief and will deal only with a few findings of special interest. Since its introduction into clinical use in 1977, demonstration of safety and efficacy by a number of investigators,[21, 23, 83, 86] and approval by the FDA in 1982, the implantable infusion pump has become widely used for the infusion of cancer chemotherapeutic agents. To date, approximately 7,000 Infusaid pumps have been implanted for this purpose.

No randomized prospective clinical trial results have been reported as yet, but Balch et al. compared the survival of 81 patients who received regional 5-FUDR infusion chemotherapy in the treatment of colorectal hepatic metastases with survival of a historical control group of 129 patients with isolated liver metastates.[87] Major prognostic indicators were similar for both groups. Carcinoembryonic antigen levels fell by one third or more after two cycles of chemotherapy in 88% of patients receiving 5-FUDR by pump. The pump group had improved 1-year (82% vs. 36%) and median (26 months vs. 8 months; $P <$ .001) survival when compared with the control group. An interesting finding of this study was that the natural course of development of the disease was changed by this treatment approach. Whereas, in the past the major cause of death was tumor progression in the liver, hepatic metastases were effectively controlled by this treatment. Progression of disease in lung or bone was the cause of death in the majority of these patients. These promising early results appear to be corroborated by the results of a similar study of 60 patients performed by Ensminger and colleagues at the University of Michigan which had a 21-month median survival in the pump group.[85] The above data await confirmation by randomized prospective trials that are now in progress.

Intraspinal Morphine

Utilization of an implantable infusion pump to deliver analgesic intrathecally or epidurally has been described in case reports and in studies of series of patients. Onofrio and associates, who initiated this technique for intrathecal morphine delivery, found they were able to achieve a pain-free state in the single patient studied, while preserving motor and sensory functions that are usually suppressed by parenteral narcotics.[24] Similar results have been described in case reports by other authors who administered morphine either intrathecally[88] or epidurally.[84, 89] Coombs et al. studied a series of 13 patients who received epidural morphine infusions from implantable pumps for periods of up to 8 months.[90] In this series, constant intraspinal flow rates of morphine were observed, with no incidence of catheter or pump infection, respiratory depression, or pump failure. Another series of ten patients with intractable pain (five with cancer and five with nonmalignant disease), were evaluated by psychometric examination after 12 weeks of epidural morphine therapy. Both groups required significant serial increases in morphine dosage over time, indicating the development of spinal opiate receptor tolerance. Sustained analgesic response was maintained in the cancer patients but response in the patients with nonmalignant disease was poor.[91] All of the above studies were performed with Infusaid pumps.

Insulin

Clinical experience with implantable insulin pumps has been reviewed in depth by Irsigler.[92] A registry for clinical studies with implantable pumps has been established by the International Study Group on Diabetes Treatment with Implantable Insulin Delivery Devices. Currently 103 implantable pumps have been placed for insulin infusion in the treatment of diabetes.[93] Of these, eight are electronically controlled peristaltic pumps; the remaining 95 are single-flow-rate Infusaid pumps.

Of the eight electronic pumps implanted, four were constructed by Sandia Laboratories and implanted by Eaton, Schade and colleagues of the University of New Mexico (Albuquerque). These four pumps were implanted in three patients (in one patient the pump was replaced after 5 months when its battery became exhausted). In the report of early results from their first patient, Schade et al. found that intraperitoneal insulin delivery from the unit normalized the patient's plasma glucose, plasma insulin, and glycosylated hemoglobin concentrations.[48]

The remaining four electronic pumps were manufactured by Siemens AG. One device was implanted by Irsigler et al., who found that it achieved near-normalization of glycemia.[53] It ultimately had to be replaced because of electronic failure after 7 months, and the replacement also failed due to catheter damage after 2 months.[81, 94]

A Siemens pump implanted by Selam et al. also achieved near normoglycemia and maintained it for 14 months with intraperitoneal insulin infusion.[63] Insulin requirements were slightly reduced, although possibly due to voluntary weight reduction by the patient. The hypoglycemic episodes, although not entirely eliminated, were always minor.

Walter's group in Munich implanted a Siemens programmable pump for IV delivery. The device was removed after 10 months because of deteriorating metabolic control in the patient.

Of the 95 Infusaid pumps that have been implanted for diabetes, 29 were implanted by our group at the University of Minnesota, 12 by Dr. Blackshear's group at Harvard University, two by Drs. Beyer, Schulz, and colleagues (Mainz), and the remaining 52 by Irsigler, Kritz, and associates of Vienna.

Our experience with a series of five type II diabetics has been reported previously.[29] In this study, mean postprandial glucose and mean fasting glucose values improved on continuous insulin infusion by pump when compared with previous regimens of insulin injections. Glycosylated hemoglobin (HbAlc) was normalized and, interestingly, C peptide became elevated over the course of time in these subjects, rising from 0.42 ± 0.33 to 0.93 ± 0.43 ng/ml ($P < .01$). Since then our patient population has expanded to include a total of 18 type II diabetics and 11 type I diabetics. None of the type II patients take any insulin other than the continuous infusion provided by the pump. Our type I diabetics generally supplement insulin provided by the pump with one or more insulin injections daily to minimize prandial glycemic excursions; however, some of these patients do not supplement their insulin by subcutaneous injections. Patient acceptance of the pumps has been high and pump performance has been excellent throughout, 3,131 patient-months of insulin infusion.

Three of the type I patients had documented peripheral insulin resistance. IV insulin from the pump has led to a substantial reduction of days of hospitalization in these patients and may have been lifesaving. After continuous IV insulin infusion was established in these individuals, they also appeared to lose their peripheral resistance to subcutaneous insulin and were able to supplement their IV insulin with subcutaneous insulin injections.

Blackshear et al. carefully studied two type II diabetics who received IV insulin from their implanted pumps.[95] They found that mean 24-hour plasma glucose levels decreased, glycosuria was eliminated, and HbAlc levels were in or near the normal range during the 1-year infusion periods. Improvements were also noted in serum triglycerides, serum anti-insulin antibody titers, and vitreous fluorescein concentrations after IV fluorescein injections. Euglycemic insulin clamp studies showed that no significant changes in glucose disposal rate occurred after treatment. However, insulin secretion was enhanced during hypoglycemic insulin clamp tests in both patients after prolonged insulin infusion. Blackshear currently is studying a total of 12 patients.

Schulz et al. studied two patients with type I diabetes and reported that the frequency of hyperglycemic and hypoglycemic episodes were decreased and that the parameters of blood glucose control (MBG, MAGE, M-value, and HbAlc) were improved by continuous intraperitoneal infusion of insulin with subcutaneous insulin injection supplements.[96]

Kritz et al. reported the results of constant rate insulin infusion in 21 patients with type I diabetes and one pancreatectomized patient.[97] The majority of these patients received insulin via the intraperitoneal route. They found that MBG levels were significantly lower on constant rate insulin infusion with supplemental injections than with insulin injections alone. Also, HbAlc values fell significantly. The frequency of hypoglycemic episodes decreased, and there was only a single recorded instance of hypoglycemic attack. Interestingly, improvement was seen in four quantifiable parameters of diabetic neuropathy when patients were on pump therapy.

The Future of Implantable Infusion Pumps

Implantable drug infusion device development is a burgeoning industry in its infancy with a vast potential to improve the quality of medical care that can be provided. Coming into being at a time when recombinant DNA technology is in a similar stage of growth, these two fields of endeavor have an opportunity to grow synergistically to produce drug and device combinations that exceed the therapeutic effects that drugs alone can provide. These technologies will be particularly important in the evolution of new peptide therapeutic agents, since genetic engineering promises to make these substances more widely available and less expensive and since implantable drug infusion devices promise to overcome several major obstacles to their use.

With respect to certain of these problems solvable by implantable infusion devices, we postulate the following. First, many peptides are highly vulnerable to gastric acid and gastrointestinal enzymes and thus are unacceptable except for parenteral delivery. Second, the therapeutic index of many such drugs is narrow and the precision of delivery required is beyond the capability of the oral route of administration. Third, the site of delivery may be important in achieving therapeutic effectiveness or avoiding side effects. For example, an active therapeutic agent for the treatment of Parkinson's disease is dopamine, which does not cross the blood-brain barrier. Thus, this disease is currently treated with oral doses of levodopa, a compound that does cross the blood-brain barrier and is converted by enzymes in the brain to dopamine. Unfortunately, intestinal bacteria also make such enzymes, so the quantity of a given oral dose that reaches the brain as levodopa is highly variable and largely uncontrollable, leading to continued impairment of motor coordination and, thus, the inability of patients to live independently. An implantable infusion pump could provide dopamine directly into the brain ventricles or, alternatively, infuse levodopa IV, thereby avoiding the influences of intestinal bacterial enzymes. Other diseases in which therapeutic success of available drugs might be improved by direct delivery across the blood-brain barrier are amyotrophic lateral sclerosis (Lou Gehrig's disease) and Alzheimer's disease.

New implantable infusion pump technology can potentially vastly expand the ability of the medical community to deal with disease. It is incumbent upon the community of medical professionals to meet this challenge and make this promise a reality.

REFERENCES

1. Deansley R., Parkes A.S.: Factors influencing the effectiveness of administered hormones. *Proc. R. Soc. London [Biol.]* 124:279, 1937.
2. Langer R., Urquhart J., Blackshear P.J.: Implantable drug delivery systems. *Trans. Am. Soc. Artif. Intern. Organs* 27:648, 1981.

3. Brown H.S., Meltzer G., Merrill R.C., et al.: Visual effects of pilocarpine in glaucoma. *Arch. Ophthalmol.* 94:1716, 1976.
4. Rybo G.: The IUD and endometrial bleeding. *J. Reprod. Med.* 20:175, 1978.
5. Rose S., Nelson J.F.: A continuous long-term injector. *Aust. J. Exp. Biol.* 33:415, 1955.
6. Theeuwes F., Yum S.I.: Principles of design and operation of generic osmotic pumps for the delivery of semisolid or liquid formulations. *Ann. Biomed. Eng.* 4:343, 1976.
7. Theeuwes F.: Elementary osmotic pump. *J. Pharm. Sci.* 64:1987, 1975.
8. Ommaya A.K.: Subcutaneous reservoir and pump for sterile access to ventricular cerebrospinal fluid. *Lancet* 2:293, 1963.
9. Smith A.N., Pershaw R.M., Bisset W.N.: The drainage of resistant ascites by a modification of the Spitz-Holter valve technique. *J. R. Col. Surg. Edinb.* 7:289, 1962.
10. Leveen H.H., Christoudias G., Moon I., et al.: Peritoneo-venous shunting for ascites. *Ann. Surg.* 180:580, 1974.
11. Lund R.H., Newkirk J.B.: Peritoneo-venous shunting system for the surgical management of ascites. *Contemp. Surg.* 14:31, 1979.
12. Summers G.D.: A new and growing family of artificial implanted fluid-control devices. *Trans. Am. Soc. Artif. Intern. Organs* 16:218, 1970.
13. Niederhuber J.E., Ensminger W., Gyves J.W., et al.: Totally implanted venous and arterial access systems to replace external catheters in cancer treatment. *Surgery* 92:706, 1982.
14. Blackshear P.J., Dorman F.D., Blackshear P.L. Jr., et al.: A permanently implantable self-recycling low flow constant rate multipurpose infusion pump of simple design. *Surg. Forum* 21:136, 1970.
15. Blackshear P.J., Dorman F.D., Blackshear P.L. Jr., et al.: The design and initial testing of an implantable infusion pump. *Surg. Gynecol. Obstet.* 134:51, 1972.
16. Blackshear P.J., Rohde, T.D., Varco R.L., et al.: One year of continuous heparinization in the dog using a totally implantable infusion pump. *Surg. Gynecol. Obstet.* 141:176, 1975.
17. Rohde T.D., Blackshear P.J., Varco R.L., et al.: One year of heparin anticoagulation in an ambulatory subject with a totally implantable pump. *Minn. Med.* 60:719, 1977.
18. Rohde T.D., Blackshear P.J., Varco R.L., et al.: Protracted parenteral drug infusion in ambulatory subjects using an implantable infusion pump. *Trans. Am. Soc. Artif. Intern. Organs* 23:13, 1977.
19. Buchwald H., Rohde T.D., Schneider P.D., et al.: Long-term continuous intravenous heparin administration by an implantable infusion pump in ambulatory patients with recurrent venous thrombosis. *Surgery* 88:507, 1980.
20. Chapleau C.E., Robertson J.T.: Spontaneous cervical carotid artery dissection: Outpatient treatment with continuous heparin infusion using a totally implantable infusion device. *Neurosurgery* 8:83, 1981.
21. Buchwald H., Grage T.B., Vassilopoulos P.P., et al.: Intra-arterial infusion chemotherapy for hepatic carcinoma using a totally implantable infusion pump. *Cancer* 45:866, 1980.

22. Cohen A.M., Wood W.C., Greenfield A., et al.: Transbrachial hepatic arterial chemotherapy using an implantable infusion pump. *Dis. Colon Rectum* 23:223, 1980.
23. Ensminger W., Niederhuber J., Dakhil S., et al.: Totally implanted drug delivery system for hepatic arterial chemotherapy. *Cancer Treat. Rep.* 65:393, 1981.
24. Onofrio B.M., Yaksh T.L., Arnold P.G.: Continuous low-dose intrathecal morphine administration in the treatment of chronic pain of malignant origin. *Mayo Clin. Proc.* 56:516, 1981.
25. Blackshear P.J., Rohde T.D., Prosl F., et al.: The implantable infusion pump: A new concept in drug delivery. *Med. Prog. Technol.* 6:149, 1979.
26. Buchwald H., Rohde T.D., Dorman F.D., et al.: A totally implantable drug infusion device: Laboratory and clinical experience using a model with single flow rate and a new design for modulated insulin infusion. *Diabetes Care* 3:351, 1980.
27. Blackshear P.J., Rohde T.D., Palmer J.L., et al.: Glycerol prevents insulin precipitation and interruption of flow in an implantable insulin infusion pump. *Diabetes Care* 6:387, 1983.
28. Buchwald H., Barbosa J.J., Varco R.L., et al.: Treatment of a type II diabetic patient by means of a totally implantable insulin infusion device. *Lancet* 8232:1233, 1981.
29. Rupp W.M., Barbosa J.J., Blackshear P.J., et al.: Improvement in blood glucose control in five adult-onset (type II) diabetic patients treated with an implantable insulin infusion device. *N. Engl. J. Med.* 307:265, 1982.
30. Kadish A.H.: Automation control of blood sugar: I. A servomechanism for glucose monitoring and control. *Am. J. Med. Electron.* 3:82, 1964.
31. Pfeiffer E.F., Thum C., Clemens A.H.: The artificial beta cell: A continuous control of blood sugar by external regulation of insulin infusion (glucose controlled insulin infusion system). *Horm. Metab. Res.* 6:339, 1974.
32. Albisser A.M., Leibel B.S., Ewart T.G., et al.: Clinical control of diabetes by artificial pancreas. *Diabetes* 23:397, 1974.
33. Soeldner J.S., Chang K.W., Aisenberg S., et al.: Progress towards an implantable glucose sensor and an artificial beta cell, in Urquhart J., Yates F.E. (eds.): *Temporal Aspects of Therapeutics.* New York, Plenum Press, 1973.
34. Chang L.W., Aisenberg S., Soeldner J.S., et al.: Validation of bioengineering aspects of an implantable glucose sensor. *Trans. Am. Soc. Artif. Intern. Organs* 352:19, 1973.
35. Clark L.C. Jr., Lyons C.: Electrode systems for continuous monitoring in cardiovascular surgery. *Ann. NY Acad. Sci.* 102:29, 1962.
36. Clark L.C. Jr.: Monitor and control of blood and tissue oxygen tensions. *Trans. Am. Soc. Artif. Intern. Organs* 2:41, 1956,
37. Updike S.J., Hicks G.P.: The enzyme electrode. *Nature* 214:986, 1967.
38. Bessman S.P., Schultz R.D.: Prototype glucose-oxydase sensor for the artificial pancreas. *Trans. Am. Soc. Artif. Intern. Organs* 19:361, 1973.
39. Thomas L.J., Bessman S.P.: Prototype for an implantable micropump powered by piezoelectric disk benders. *Trans. Am. Soc. Artif. Intern. Organs* 21:516, 1975.

40. Bessman S.P., Hellyer J.M., Layne E.C., et al.: The total implantation of an artificial B-cell in a dog: Progress report. International Congress Series, Amsterdam, Excerpta Medica, 1977, vol. 413, p. 496.
41. Slama C., Hautecouverture M., Assan R., et al.: One to five days of continuous intravenous insulin infusion in seven diabetic patients. Diabetes 23:732, 1974.
42. Pickup J.C., Keen H., Parsons J.A., et al.: Continuous subcutaneous insulin infusion: An approach to achieving normoglycemia. Br. Med. J. 1:204, 1978.
43. Tamborlane W.V., Sherwin R.S., Genel M., et al.: Reduction to normal of plasma glucose in juvenile diabetes by subcutaneous administration of insulin with a portable infusion pump. N. Engl. J. Med. 300:573, 1979.
44. Shumakov V.I.: Discussion, in Thomas L.J., Bessman S.P.: Prototype for an implantable micropump powered by piezoelectric disk benders. Trans. Am. Soc. Artif. Intern. Organs 21:516, 1975.
45. Spencer W.J., Corbett W.T.: Dominquez L.R., et al.: An electronically controlled piezoelectric insulin pump and valves. IEEE Trans. SU-25:153, 1978.
46. Spencer W.J.: For diabetics: An electronic pancreas. IEEE Spectrum June 1978, p. 38.
47. Carlson G.A., Love J.T., Urenda R.S., et al.: Development of an artificial beta cell suitable for animal implantation. Trans. Am. Soc. Artif. Intern. Organs 26:523, 1980.
48. Schade D.S., Eaton R.P., Edwards W.S., et al.: A remotely programmable insulin delivery system: Successful short-term implantation in man. JAMA 247:1848, 1982.
49. Hepp K.D., Renner R., von Funcke H.J., et al.: Glucose homeostasis under continuous intravenous insulin therapy in diabetics. Horm. Metab. Res. Suppl. 7:72, 1977.
50. Irsigler K., Kritz H.: Long-term continuous intravenous insulin therapy with a portable insulin dosage-regulating apparatus. Diabetes 28:196, 1979.
51. Froesch E.R., B.atter G., Morell B.: Optimal blood sugar control in labile diabetics using a portable open-loop insulin infusion system with a flexible program. Horm. Metab. Res. 8:198, 1979.
52. Prestele K., Franetzki M., Kresse H.: Development of program-controlled portable insulin delivery devices. Diabetes Care 3:362, 1980.
53. Irsigler K., Kritz H., Hagmuller G., et al.: Long-term continuous intraperitoneal insulin infusion with an implanted remote-controlled insulin infusion device. Diabetes 30:1072, 1981.
54. Dorman F.D., Rohde T.D., Arlt G.J., et al.: A two-phase fluid powered insulin infusion pump with basal-bolus capability which compensates for pressure and temperature variability. Trans. Am. Soc. Artif. Intern. Organs 27:236, 1981.
55. Perkins P.R., Dorman F.D., Rohde T.D., et al.: Design and initial testing of a totally implantable transcutaneously controllable insulin delivery device. Trans. Am. Soc. Artif. Intern. Organs 24:229, 1978.
56. Rohde T.D., Wigness B.D., Dorman F.D., et al.: Glucoregulation in the

dog by implantable pump and conventional means. *Trans. Am. Soc. Artif. Intern. Organs* 28:249, 1982.

57. Rhode T.D., Wigness B.D., Rupp W.M., et al.: Control of glycemia in four routes of insulin administration in diabetic dogs. *Trans. Am. Soc. Artif. Intern. Organs* 29:720, 1983.

58. Watkins E.: Chronometric Infuser: An apparatus for protocol ambulatory infusion therapy. *N. Engl. J. Med.* 269:850, 1963.

59. Carlson G.A., Blair R.E., Gaona J.I. Jr., et al.: An implantable remotely programmable insulin infusion system. *Sandia Report SAND* 81:2152, 1981.

60. Zingg W., Unger F.: Reports from representatives of industry, in Irsigler K., Kritz H., Lovett R. (eds.): *Diabetes Treatment With Implantable Insulin Infusion Systems*. Vienna, Urban & Schwarzenberg, 1983, p. 29.

61. Greatbatch W.: Engineering and instrumentation in the manufacture and patient delivery of drugs. *Med. Instrum.* 17:9, 1983.

62. Selam J.L., Slingenmeyer A., Chaptal P.A., et al.: Total implantation of a remotely controlled insulin minipump in a human insulin-dependent diabetic. *Artif. Organs* 6:315, 1982.

63. Selam J.L., Slingenmeyer A., Chaptal P.A., et al.: One year continuous run with a totally implantable Siemens Pump in a human diabetic, in Irsigler K., Kritz H., Lovett R. (eds.): *Diabetes Treatment With Implantable Insulin Infusion Systems*. Vienna, Urban & Schwarzenberg, 1983, p. 119.

64. Comben R., Bartelt K., Elsberry D., et al.: Experimental and clinical studies using Medtronic's programmable implantable drug administration device. *Artif. Organs* 7A:107, 1983.

65. Comben R., Penn R., Bartelt K., et al.: A multi-pourpose implantable drug administration system. Read before the International Workshop on Insulin and Portable Delivery Devices, Toronto, June 9–11, 1982.

66. Saudek C.D., Fischell R.E.: The achievement of normoglycemia by use of a programmable, implantable medication system. Read before the International Workshop on Insulin and Portable Delivery Devices, Toronto, June 9–11, 1982.

67. Fischell R.E., Radford W.E., Hogrefe A.F., et al.: A programmable implantable system (PIMS) for the treatment of diabetes. *Artif. Organs* 7A:82, 1983.

68. Bessman S.P., Thomas L.J., Kojima H., et al.: The implantation of a closed loop artificial beta cell in dogs. *Trans. Am. Soc. Artif. Intern. Organs* 27:7, 1981.

69. Schubert W., Baurschmidt P., Nagol J., et al.: An implantable artificial pancreas. *Med. Biol. Eng. Comput.* 18:527, 1980.

70. Sefton M.V., Lusher H.M., Firth S.R., et al.: Controlled release micropump for insulin administration. *Ann. Biomed. Eng.* 7:329, 1979.

71. Sefton M.V., Horvath V., Allen D.G., et al.: Insulin delivery from an implantable controlled release micropump in pancreatectomized dogs. *Trans. Am. Soc. Artif. Intern. Organs* 29:714, 1983.

72. NIH Publication No. 80-2073. Bethesda, Md., 1973.

73. Blackshear P.J., Rohde T.D.: Artificial devices for insulin infusion in the

treatment of patients with diabetes mellitus, in Bruck S.D. (ed.): Controlled Drug Delivery: vol. II, Clinical Applications. Boca Raton, CRC Press, 1983.

74. Lougheed W.D., Woulfe-Flanagan H., Clement J.R., et al.: Insulin aggregation in artificial delivery systems. Diabetologia 19:1, 1980.

75. Insulin Delivery Workshop Report to National Diabetes Advisory Board. Second National Conference on Diabetes, Reston, Va., Sept. 25–28, 1983.

76. Buchwald H.: Implantation for infusion into the superior vena cava, in Irsigler K., Kritz H., Lovett R. (eds.): Diabetes Treatment With Implantable Infusion Systems. Vienna, Urban & Schwarzenberg, 1983, p. 276.

77. Hagmueller G.W.: Surgical techniques of pump implantation, in Irsigler K., Kirtz H., Lovett R. (eds.): Diabetes Treatment With Implantable Insulin Infusion Systems. Vienna, Urban & Schwarzenberg, 1983, p. 277.

78. Diagnostic and therapeutic technology assessment (DATTA): Implantable infusion pump. JAMA 250:1906, 1983.

79. Kinney E.L., Allen R.P., Weidner W.A., et al.: Recurrent pulmonary emboli secondary to right atrial thrombus around a permanent pacing catheter: A case report and review of the literature. Pace 2:196, 1979.

80. Fabri P.J., Mirallo J.M., Ruberg R.L., et al.: Incidence and prevention of thrombosis of the subclavian vein during total parenteral nutrition. Surg. Gynecol. Obstet. 155:238, 1982.

81. Kritz H., Najemnik C., Hagmueller G., et al.: Long-term results using different routes of insulin infusion, in Irsigler K., Kritz H., Lovett R. (eds.): Diabetes Treatment With Implantable Infusion Systems. Vienna, Urban & Schwarzenberg, 1983, p. 81.

82. Watkins E., Sullivan R.D.: Cancer chemotherapy by prolonged arterial infusion. Surg. Gynecol. Obstet. 118:3, 1964.

83. Cohen A.M., Greenfield A., Wood W.C., et al.: Treatment of hepatic metastases by transaxillary hepatic artery chemotherapy using an implanted drug pump. Cancer 51:2013, 1983.

84. Harbaugh R.E., Coombs D.W., Saunders R.L., et al.: Implanted continuous epidural morphine infusion system. J. Neurosurg. 56:803, 1982.

85. Chute E., Buchwald H.: Chemotherapy with a totally implantable infusion pump, unpublished manuscript.

86. Barone R.M., Byfeld J.E., Goldfarb P.B., et al.: Intra-arterial chemotherapy using an inplantable infusion pump and liver radiation for the treatment of hepatic metastases. Cancer 50:850, 1982.

87. Balch C.M., Urist M.M., Soong S., et al.: A prospective phase II clinical trial of continuous FUDR regional chemotherapy for colorectal metastases of the liver using a totally implantable drug infusion pump. Ann. Surg. 198:567, 1983.

88. Greenberg H.S., Taren J., Ensminger W.D., et al.: Benefit from and tolerance to continued intrathecal infusion of morphine for intractable cancer pain. J. Neurosurg. 57:360, 1982.

89. Coombs D.W., Saunders R.L., Pageau M.G.: Continuous intraspinal narcotic analgesia: Technical aspects of an implantable infusion system. Reg. Anaesth. 7:100, 1982.

90. Coombs D.W., Saunders R.L., Gaylor M., et al.: Epidural narcotic infu-

sion reservoir: Implantation technique and efficacy. *Anesthesiology* 56:469, 1982.

91. Coombs D.W., Saunders R.L., Gaylor M.S., et al.: Relief of continuous chronic pain by intraspinal narcotic infusion via an implantable reservoir. *JAMA* 250:2336, 1983.

92. Irsigler K.: Keynote address, second ISGIID meeting, January 1983, in Irsigler K., Kritz H., Lovett R. (eds.): *Diabetes Treatment With Implantable Insulin Infusion Systems.* Vienna, Urban & Schwarzenberg, 1983, p. 1.

93. Irsigler K., Kritz H., Bali C.: *Newsletter,* International Study Group on Diabetes Treatment With Implantable Insulin Delivery Devices, November 1983.

94. Knatterud G.L.: First report of the status of the ISGIID Register in Irsigler K., Kritz H., Lovett R. (eds.): *Diabetes Treatment With Implantable Insulin Infusion Systems.* Vienna, Urban & Schwarzenberg, 1983, p. 7.

95. Blackshear P.J., Shulman G.I., Nathan D.M., et al.: Metabolic response to one year of continuous, basal rate intravenous insulin infusion in type II diabetic patients, unpublished manuscript.

96. Schulz G., Beyer M., Hogan M., et al.: Implantable insulin infusion devices in the therapy of type I diabetes, in Irsigler K., Kritz H., Lovett R. (eds.): *Diabetes Treatment With Implantable Insulin Infusion Systems.* Vienna, Urban & Schwarzenberg, 1983, p. 12.

97. Kritz H., Hagmueller G., Lovett R., et al.: Implantable constant basal rate insulin infusion devices for Type I (insulin-dependent) diabetic patients. *Diabetologia* 25:78, 1983.

Complications of Gastric Partitioning for Morbid Obesity

JUAN BASS, M.D. AND JOEL B. FREEMAN, M.D.,
FRCS(c), FACS

From the Division of General Surgery, University of Ottawa, Ottawa General
Hospital, Ottawa, Ontario, Canada.

OBESITY is a serious nutritional disorder which affects one third of the North American population. Nearly 5% of North Americans weigh more than twice their ideal weight, corrected for age, sex, and height. Patients who are 30% over their ideal weight have an increased risk of early death, which rises in direct proportion to excess weight.[1-5] Morbid obesity contributes significantly to an increased morbidity and mortality associated with such conditions as heart disease, hypertension, abnormalities of lipid metabolism, diabetes, arthritis, pulmonary insufficiency, and susceptibility to operative complications when such patients require surgery.[6-8] The medical treatment of morbid obesity, including diets, group therapy, behavior modification, and expensive luxury clinics or camps, results in significant and sustained weight loss of 40 lb in less than 5% of patients.[9-11] Spectacular claims for weight loss by conservative treatment, particularly for the morbidly obese, are seldom if ever substantiated by long-term follow-up data. A recent NIH Consensus Forum confirmed the inadequacy and incomplete follow-up data of most weight loss groups in America.[12]

Many obese patients live as social recluses, isolating themselves from family and society. Travel may be impossible due

0065-3411/84/0018-0223-0256-$04.00

to pain, exertional dyspnea, or inability to fit into the transportation seat.

The Framingham Study documented the beneficial effects of weight loss with respect to blood pressure, plasma lipid levels, uric acid, and glucose tolerance.[13] This study also indicated that coronary artery disease would decrease by 25% and cerebral infarction by 35% if all patients in the study were at normal weight. Other benefits include frequent amelioration of hypertension, a decrease in the incidence of gallstones, reversal of cardiorespiratory impairment(s), reduction of hypertriglyceridemia and hypercholesterolemia, elevated high-density lipoprotein levels, and improved or even complete normalization of abnormal glucose tolerance, improved cardiovascular fitness and ability to exercise, an improvement in arthritis related to excess weight, better surgical results when reconstructive joint surgery is required, and psychosocial rehabilitation. Obesity acquired between the ages of 20–40 years may have a much greater effect on the development of subsequent cardiovascular disease than obesity acquired after the age of 40.[3] Similarly, the middle-aged, hypertensive, overweight, male smoker is at greater risk than his normotensive, nonsmoking female counterpart.[3] Undoubtedly, there are "benign" forms of obesity in which the patient's only problem is the extra weight.

The indications for surgical intervention are well established. What is problematic is how to choose the compliant patient who will adapt to the many life style changes required for long-term success. Surgery should not be considered in patients less than twice ideal body weight corrected for height. There must be a clear history of repeated, failed attempts at weight loss by well-controlled conservative measures and the patient must have been morbidly obese for at least 5 years with no evidence of organic etiology. Patients over 45 do not tolerate surgical complications well and they cannot change life style. The risks of surgery combined with poor results are relative contraindications to surgery over the age of 45.[15] Serious medical problems may be indications or contraindications to surgery. For example, crippling arthritis and insulin-dependent diabetes in a 50-year-old patient may sway the surgeon toward operative treatment. Conversely, a duodenal ulcer, inflammatory bowel disease, severe renal or hepatic dysfunction, alcoholism, and overt psychoses are contraindications. Evidence of impulsive behavior wherein the patient requests operation immediately calls for caution. Such patients are looking for quick cures and will not change eating habits or participate in exercise programs. If patients will not submit to an intensive (3–6 month) education process in an obesity clinic, they will probably not sustain weight loss. The psychiatric assessment may give an indication of the patient's compliance and it rules out psychotic or severe neurotic disorders. The patient must have a clear understanding of the risks and complications of the operation and the postoperative dietary restrictions. Most centers use educational booklets or audiovisual programs and arrange meetings with patients who have had the procedure. Separate consent forms clearly delineating the risk-benefit aspects of the operation should be read and preferably signed, in addition to the regular surgical consent form.

Given the frequency of obesity, its associated risks of death and morbidity, and the high level of physician frustration in dealing with this disese, surgeons have been increasingly called on to treat such patients, who may be slowly dying from their disease. The history of surgical treatment for morbid obesity covers nearly two decades and many operations. Essential is that each operation gained wide acceptance before 2-year evaluation. Reviews of the various surgical treatments are available elsewhere.[16–18] The remainder of this chapter will address the complications and long-term results of gastric partitioning operations for morbid obesity, which can be broadly classified as follows: gastric bypass (GBP) with loop gastrojejunostomy, GBP with Roux-en-Y gastrojejunostomy, GBP with Silastic reinforcement, biliary enteric bypass, horizontal gastroplasty (HGP), vertical banded gastroplasty (VBG), and gastric wrap.

GBP with loop gastrojejunostomy was the first procedure done by Mason, and Ito in 1967.[19] Initially the stomach was completely divided, but this technique was subsequently simplified by the introduction of stapling instruments which partitioned rather than divided the stomach. This operation is still practiced, although most surgeons agree that a Roux-en-Y anastomosis between the stomach and intestine is preferable. This avoids bile reflux and improves drainage of the distal gastric pouch. GBP was performed from 1968 until 1972, when a number of surgeons proposed that nearly complete partitioning of the stomach, leaving a narrow greater curve channel, would be equally efficacious while avoiding the dangers of a gastrojejunal anastomosis. This was followed by a virtual explosion of HGP techniques as more and more centers took up the operation. With GBP, risks were great and operating time was long, but with the advent of HGP, the scope of the operation fell well within the technical capabilities of many surgeons. HGP was never equal to GBP in the short run, and in the longer term, failure rates escalated to the point where it has basically been abandoned.[20, 21] Perhaps all bariatric surgeons would have reverted to GBP if it were not for the development of the VBG, again by Mason.[22] This procedure creates a lesser curve channel, which, along with excision of a window of the anterior and posterior gastric walls with the EEA stapler, permits a completely reinforced channel. All previous GP stomas, located either in the center or on the greater curve of the stomach, could not be reinforced 360 degrees.

Flanagan developed a GBP wherein the anastomosis was reinforced by a Silastic ring in an attempt to prevent stoma dilation. Early results are encouraging but long-term data are needed.[23] Wilkinson developed a restrictive operation wherein the entire stomach is wrapped in a sheet of Marlex. This operation is attractive because of its apparent simplicity and because the stomach is not entered. Again, long-term data are anxiously awaited. The biliary enteric bypass is a third operation which has been studied in Europe, with some early North American data beginning to appear.[24] The latter two operations will not be discussed further in this review.

Anesthetic Considerations

Morbid obesity is a challenge to the anesthesiologist. Simple procedures such as starting an intravenous line may prove difficult and time-consuming. We insert a subclavian catheter the day before surgery and a chest x-ray film is obtained to confirm position and verify the absence of pneumothorax. This may save 20 minutes of operating room time. Positive pressure ventilation may convert a small asymptomatic pneumothorax into a significant one. Insertion of central lines immediately prior to surgery should be via the external or internal jugular veins, as these routes are rarely associated with pneumothorax. Airway management is more difficult in these patients. The thick anterior wall may interfere with placement of the laryngoscope handle, and obtaining a good fit with the mask may be impossible. Placement of radial artery catheters or any regional anesthetic procedure is made more difficult by the absence of bony landmarks and the longer distance to the target. If adequate time has not been allowed for preparation of these patients, long delays add to the frustration of all those concerned.

Hypoxemia may exist preoperatively and can worsen substantially during and after surgery.[25–28] General anesthesia itself, regardless of technique, is associated with a further diminution of lung volumes. Hence, all patients must have arterial blood gases and pulmonary function analyzed preoperatively. Patients should also have arterial blood gas values measured intraoperatively via an arterial line. Blood pressure monitoring by cuff is notoriously inaccurate in the morbidly obese patient, particularly if an extra-large cuff is not used. This is a second indication for the arterial line.[29]

Morbidly obese patients have large anatomical shunts plus ventilation-perfusion inequalities, both at rest and during exercise.[27] The major defect is anatomical: increased weight on the abdominal wall produces kyphosis and decreased chest expansion, while the increased chest wall thickness itself contributes to impaired chest wall compliance. Hypoventilation and reductions in chest wall compliance, particularly in the recumbent position, complicate postoperative ventilation. A reduced functional residual capacity (FRC) is the most common pulmonary function abnormality noted in obesity. This is caused by a reduction in the expiratory reserve volume so that closing capacity exceeds FRC during tidal breathing.[30] These changes are accentuated in the supine position but may be present in the sitting position in the superheavyweights, emphasizing the importance of ambulation and avoidance of bed rest. Pulmonary artery pressure increases by 31% and pulmonary arterial wedge pressure by 44% in the supine versus sitting positions. Proper fluid management is critical in such patients, in whom fluid overload is poorly tolerated.

The risk of aspiration is greater in obese patients than in controls because of larger residual gastric volumes and low pH.[28] All upper abdominal operations done through midline incisions result in a greater incidence of atelectasis, and this is more pronounced in the morbidly obese.[31] There is a more significant and prolonged reduction in arterial Po_2 with vertical as opposed to transverse incisions.

Pulmonary embolism has not been a major problem in our 7 years of experience with gastric partitioning, in that no major emboli have been documented. We do not use subcutaneous heparin unless there is a history of previous emboli, phlebitis, or cardiac disease. However, others use subcutaneous heparin routinely. We have been unable to find evidence in the literature which documents that the incidence of pulmonary emboli is higher in the morbidly obese. All patients should have antiembolic stockings, and 5% dextrose should be infused for at least 12 hours preoperatively to reduce serum fatty acid levels, which are thrombogenic.[33] The operating table is placed in the reverse Trendelenburg position intermittently during surgery, and early ambulation is emphasized.

Pulmonary parenchymal compliance may be normal or reduced by 10%–20% in simple obesity and by as much as 40% in the obesity-hypoventilation syndrome.[25] In the latter condition there is an increase in the pulmonary extravascular water. Chest wall compliance is reduced markedly in the obesity-hypoventilation syndrome and there is an increase in pulmonary blood flow volume.

Liver morphology and function are not always normal in morbidly obese patients, and one should assume that the liver's ability to tolerate stressful insults is impaired. Hence, it is important to avoid hypoxemia and hypotension.[26] Halothane metabolism is impaired.[27]

Randall et al. found no difference in the 24-hour outcome when comparing different anesthetic techniques.[28] Although many have recommended epidural or spinal anesthesia, little has been done to affirm the efficacy of such in obese patients. Fox et al. studied two groups of morbidly obese patients whose analgesia was controlled conventionally with narcotics or by extradural spinal catheters.[31] There was little difference in postoperative blood gas measurements but there was less lung collapse in the patients with extradural catheters (18.5% vs. 27.5%).

Respiratory insufficiency is rare after bariatric surgery and postoperative ventilatory or ICU support is seldom indicated. Several aspects of preoperative and postoperative care will lessen the chances of significant pulmonary complications. All patients who smoke must be encouraged to reduce the number of cigarettes to a maximum of three daily for at least 4 weeks preoperatively, and such patients are admitted 2 days prior to surgery for chest physiotherapy and incentive spirometry. Important tests include preoperative and intraoperative blood gas monitoring, preoperative pulmonary function testing, and identification of the high-risk patient with hypoxemia, sleep apnea, or CO_2 retention, who indeed may be a candidate for ICU monitoring postoperatively. We emphasize early ambulation, which begins in the recovery room 2 hours after surgery. The patient is given 5 mg of IV morphine and made to walk by the side of the bed. This is repeated at least three more times on the day of surgery. The supine position decreases FRC in all people. We keep obese patients in a 30-degree reverse Trendelenburg position intraoperatively and postoperatively. This reduces the massive weight load on the lungs and improves oxygenation. Small frequent doses of narcotics are superior to large doses, which sedate the patient and predispose to atelectasis with hypoxemia. MacLean has recommended the use of Methadone, which has a long duration of action and greatly facilitates early postoperative ambulation (personal communication). Deep breathing exercises and chest physiotherapy are helpful postoperatively and should be timed with the low-dose narcotic injections so that the patient can cough rather than sleep during the pain-free period.

The development of pneumonia, pulmonary effusions, or atelectasis suggests sepsis rather than a primary lung condition. Obese patients develop respiratory failure during sepsis because they cannot tolerate the increased respiratory demands of the hypermetabolic state. Immediate steps must be taken to rule out the possibility of a leak or other sources of sepsis. Such patients will usually require mechanical ventilation to decrease the work of respiration, but this requirement is temporary and should not last more than 48 hours after reoperation.

Postsurgical Complications

WOUND INFECTIONS

The incidence of wound infection after gastric operations for morbid obesity varies from 1.3% to 14%.[17, 33, 34] The Iowa group found the highest (14%) incidence, but this was early in their experience. The responsible organisms corresponded to those cultured from the stomach. The incidence is higher after GBP than after HGP because the stomach is opened and the nasogastric tube is often exposed to the operative area. Infection is higher after GBP than after gastric operations for peptic ulcer, perhaps reflecting the inherent disposition of the morbidly obese to wound infections.

Fat is an avascular tissue, and we adhere to the principle of avulsing rather than cutting the fat to reach the linea alba. This avoids hematomas and facilitates accurate closure. Subcutaneous sutures are avoided during abdominal closure. Paries et al. reduced wound infection from 21% to 4% with prophylactic cephazolin.[35] Irrigation of the abdominal cavity with or without antibiotics and vigorous irrigation plus abrasion of the subcutaneous tissues prior to closure are recommended. We use clips rather than sutures on the skin. With the above techniques, our wound infection rate is less than 1%.

The diagnosis of wound infections may not be easy in morbidly obese patients. A high index of suspicion is required. Fever, leukocytosis, and tachycardia may herald a simple infection or sepsis secondary to a leak. Pain, induration, or fluctuance of the wound may not be obvious, and needle aspiration or wound exploration may be indicated, even though the usual signs of infection are not present.[33]

INCISIONAL HERNIAS

The factors to be considered in the development of incisional hernias include the presence of obesity itself, age, type of incision, hematoma formation, infection, suture material, and closure technique. Mason found abdominal wall hernias in 14% of his patients at the time of GBP, confirming that obesity places an increased stress on the abdominal wall. Incisional hernias in general, and umbilical hernias specifically, may be even more common. We routinely check all patients preoperatively in the upright and supine positions using straight leg raising. Small recurrent or primary umbilical hernias should be repaired at the time of gastric partitioning, by simple incorporation into the planned incision. All umbilical hernias contain a nubbin of fat which must be removed. Larger, more complicated hernias should be repaired after appropriate weight loss, ideally at the time of panniculectomy. Larger hernias should be repaired only if the surgeon is confident that right of domain has not been lost. Otherwise, severe postoperative respiratory embarrassment may occur. Such hernia repairs may need to be deferred and then done after preoperative peritoneal air insufflation and, one hopes, after successful weight loss. Although age has no influence on the incidence of wound infections, there is a direct relationship between age and the incidence of hernia.[33] Wound infection is probably the most important etiologic factor. Mason found that 21% of patients with wound infections developed hernia, compared with only 3.5% of those without infections. Transverse incisions as were used routinely for intestinal bypass are considered stronger than vertical incisions. Some authors still use them for gastric partitioning, but most use vertical upper midline incisions. One should avoid extending the incision past the umbilicus, but this will limit the exposure, particularly in superheavyweights or those with narrow costal margins. During closure the fascial sutures should be applied at least 3 cm from the edge to avoid pull-through. The debate of whether to close with running versus interrupted sutures remains unresolved. We insert several interrupted sutures at the upper and lower ends of the wound and then complete closure with short running sutures of No. 1 Prolene or No. 2 Tvedek. Of more importance is accurate visualization of the fascia so that each bite incorporates adequate amounts of strong white tissue. Since wound infections predispose to wound hernia, subcutaneous sutures are avoided. They act as foreign bodies which devascularize without strengthening the wound. Large dead spaces or potential hematomas are treated by 48 hours of subcutaneous suction drainage.

METABOLIC AND NUTRITIONAL COMPLICATIONS

The many metabolic abnormalities which occurred after jejunoileal bypass led to its abandonment. For the first decade of their development, the most appealing feature of gastric partitioning operations was freedom from metabolic complications. However, with improved follow-up and the vast increase in the numbers of procedures being performed, metabolic and nutritional complications began to appear. The majority are due to malnutrition from excess weight loss superimposed on the preexisting obesity.

LIVER.—Liver injury, fatty metamorphosis, and infiltration

by a hyaline-like material similar to that found in alcoholic hepatitis have been described in obesity and are assumed to be due to malnutrition.[36] However, Mason et al. had only one patient with significant liver damage in 490 gastric operations, and this patient may have had halothane hepatitis.[37] Buckwalter found no progression of fatty metamorphosis 1 year postoperatively in 17 patients who underwent GBP.[38] Abnormal liver function tests have also been reported anecdotally in patients with excessive weight losses over short periods of time. Many of these were patients with post-GBP stenoses whose nutritional support was not closely supervised.[43]

NEUROLOGIC.—Memory loss and confusion with peripheral neuropathy have been encountered after gastric partitioning, usually in association with excessive weight loss.[39] Feit et al. described a patient with sensory ataxia whose postmortem examination showed extensive accumulation of lipid in the nerve cell bodies and Schwann cells suggestive of marked fat catabolism.[40] A Wernicke-Korsakoff syndrome with encephalopathy was found in another patient. Postmortem examination of the mammillary bodies was typical of the disease.[41] Several other patients have also been described, both in the literature and anecdotally at meetings.[42] These patients present with peripheral neuropathy and leg weakness, which may or may not respond to parenteral thiamine. MacLean suggested that the requirement for vitamin B complexes may be higher than formerly believed for the gastric partitioned patient losing weight rapidly.[44] Clearly, waiting for the syndrome to develop is unwise since the lesion is not always reversible, and our impression from "corridor talk" at meetings is that the problem may be more frequent than is commonly appreciated.

Brachial plexus injuries can be caused by applying excessive tension on the arms, particularly if they are suspended from IV poles to facilitate placement of the retractor. The arms should be hung with the table in its lowest position to prevent this complication. Electrical burns may also occur if the arms, or any part of the body, come into contact with the metal parts of the retractor. All of these areas must be padded.

HEMATOLOGIC.—Iron deficiency anemia is well recognized after GBP, presumably because ingested food bypasses to the duodenum. This is easily treated with oral iron supplementation. This type of anemia has not been reported after GP. Vitamin B12 and folic acid deficiency anemias have been reported after GBP.[45] If serum B12 levels are low, a Schilling test should be performed to determine if the etiology is due to poor intake or inadequate intrinsic factor. All patients having gastric partitioning of any kind should have routine periodic follow-up examinations, including a complete blood cell count and determination of serum iron level, total iron-binding capacity, B12 level, and folic acid level, in addition to liver function tests. All patients must receive multiple vitamin supplementation during the first 12–18 months when weight loss is the greatest.

RARE DEFICIENCY SYNDROMES.—Schneider et al. described a patient with stoma obstruction who developed severe malnutrition with bone marrow depression, impaired cutaneous reactivity, and other immunologic deficiencies that were reversed by parenteral nutrition.[46] Many similar cases have been discussed at meetings but never reported. When immunologic disorders develop in a patient with sepsis, chronic gastric fistula, or stoma obstruction, death can result even if the surgical complications are corrected.

Practically all patients experience some hair loss. This is attributed to either zinc deficiency or a lack of sulfur-containing amino acids. Hair loss is maximal during the first 8–12 months and always reversible.

Regardless of the type of malnutrition, prompt recognition before irreversible vitamin or immunologic changes occur is vital. Patients at greatest risk are those with stenosis, intermittent vomiting, and excessive weight loss over a short period of time. They require readmission for parenteral nutrition and correction of the underlying problem. We have routinely used feeding jejunostomies over the past 6 years. This greatly facilitates management of such patients out of the hospital and eliminates any sense of urgency for reoperation.

LEAKS

The incidence of leaks ranges from 2.5% to 6%, although some recent authors are reporting rates of less than 1% with VBG.[47, 48] Leaks were more common with the original GBP, wherein the stomach was completely divided and leaks could occur not only from the anastomosis but also from the two suture lines. Another disadvantage of GBP is that obstruction of the afferent jejunal loop can result in massive dilation of the jejunum and stomach, the pylorus acting as a one-way valve. Since the distal stomach pouch is excluded, perforation cannot be diagnosed radiologically, and reoperation must be based on visualization of massive air accumulation and clinical acumen. Proper placement and maintenance of a nasogastric tube placed through the gastrojejunostomy and into the afferent limb may prevent this problem. Extra holes must be cut so that the proximal pouch is also decompressed. The position of the tube should be confirmed prior to closure, for its tip may press on the anterior gastric wall and produce a bullet hole–type of perforation. Polyvinyl tubes harden with time. They should be removed within 48–72 hours. Others have routinely used a gastrostomy to decompress the distal pouch. The Roux-en-Y GBP eliminates this problem (provided that the Roux loop is not kinked), since the stomach is decompressed by the Roux loop into the efferent limb. Some authors use a gastrostomy tube even with this operation.

All gastric partitioning procedures are ischemic in that vessels are ligated, especially along the greater curve, and then staples are applied across the stomach with or without the application of foreign materials to prevent stoma dilation. Staple lines should be either 0.5 cm or more than 2 cm apart.[49] We have shown in dogs that incorporation of foreign material such as Marlex into the staple line around the stoma will increase the likelihood of leaks.[50] The more short gastrics that are taken, the greater the chance of leaks.[51] One should never take the left gastric or any vessels on the lesser curve. There is a posterior gastric vessel which runs from pancreas to posterior gastric wall and must be avoided during GP procedures. There is little or no danger of ischemia when VBG is performed on the lesser curve, even with Marlex, as long as vessels are not ligated. The surgeon must use his left index finger to clear fat from the posterior wall. The EEA must be carefully inserted and fired, with care taken to ensure that the hole in the stomach is circumferentially surrounded by the anvil. When the staple line is inspected from the anterior surface, one will see complete staples, but this does not necessarily mean that these staples are completely closed posteriorly. Hence, we always rotate the stomach to examine its posterior surface. Two complete donuts at least 2 mm in width must be found or a leak may occur. If there is any question, the EEA staple line is oversewn with a No. 000 nonabsorbable suture and a tongue of omentum is placed through the window. A gastrostomy tube is optional in such cases.

If desired, the anesthesiologist can infuse a mixture of 5 ml of methylene blue in 500 ml of Ringers' lactate through the nasogastric tube. The surgeon twists a penrose drain around the esophagogastric junction, but unless all of the holes in the nasogastric tube are below the penrose drain, troublesome regurgitation into the esophagus will occur without adequate distention of the pouch. This procedure may reveal unsuspected leaks. Alternatively, the EEA staple line can be submerged in sterile saline while the anesthesiologist injects air or methylene blue. IV fluorescein has been used to detect ischemic areas. The dye is injected IV, and with the overhead lights out, the stomach is examined under a Wood ultraviolet light.

As experience with HGP increased, patients began to return with poor or inadequate weight loss. Surgeons then invented increasingly aggressive techniques for preventing stoma dilation. This in turn produced more ischemia and, accordingly, more leaks or obstructions. It is interesting that many surgeons noted more complications with the "simpler" gastroplasty procedures than with GBP.

Leaks may also occur in the distal stomach either from surgical misadventure such as incorporation of a portion of the gastric wall in a closing suture or from the gastrostomy tube. The latter should be fixed with a Vicryl rather than a chromic suture. We have observed patients in whom the gastrostomy tube migrated significantly despite adequate positioning and fixation (with chromic) only days before. Also, a long (4–5 cm) Witzel tunnel should be fashioned with nonabsorbable sutures. The stomach should be fixed to the parietal peritoneum, but this is not essential. If the stomach is sutured to the parietal peritoneum under tension, the gastrostomy tube may be pulled out so that the first hole lies outside of the gastric lumen.

Next to prevention, the diagnosis of leaks is of paramount importance. Delays in diagnosis are the primary cause of mortality. Mason has clearly shown that early recognition and reoperation is the key to recovery with minimum mortality.[33, 48] Clinical recognition of sepsis in obese patients can be very difficult. Abdominal pain is rare, and frequently such patients may appear to be perfectly well, in fact asking to be discharged. Neither fever of 38.0°C nor leukocytosis over 12,000 should be present after the first 48 hours. Mason has emphasized the importance of tachycardia as a sign of early sepsis. Because of hypoxia and the subsequent hyperventilation of early sepsis, such patients may appear anxious, with flushed cheeks and slight tachypnea. Even if the chest radiograph demonstrates atelectasis, pneumonia, or pleural effusion, one should search for an intra-abdominal source. Similarly, pulmonary emboli are uncommon in these patients. Hypoxia, pulmonary consolidation, and respiratory insufficiency more often indicate sepsis. Many series report patients presumed to have died from pulmonary emboli that were, in fact, undiagnosed gastric leaks.

Other useful signs include abdominal pain, shoulder tip pain (especially in the recumbent position), back pain, and dysuria, diarrhea, or vaginal pain due to peritoneal irritation. The complaints are often nonspecific and remarkable easy to overlook.[48] Glucose intolerance, especially if the patient is receiving IV dextrose, may herald sepsis, as has been reported during parenteral nutrition. The absence of ketone production due to an inhibition of ketogenesis is well recognized during sepsis.[52]

When clinical suspicion is high, the patient should be immediately taken to the radiology suite after specimens have been obtained for culture from all appropriate sites. High-quality upright chest and abdominal films are obtained when the surgeon is in the room working with a radiologist who is both interested and experienced in interpreting postoperative GP films in morbidly obese patients. The radiographic interpretation of gastric pouches postoperatively can be difficult, and this may lead to delays in diagnosis. Air bubbles (the "soapsuds" sign) or air-fluid levels may suggest an intra-abdominal abscess, or free air may be seen. Under the fluoroscope, both diaphragms can be examined for evidence of subphrenic collections. Subphrenic collections are leaks until proved otherwise. The patient drinks a water-soluble contrast material and its course is followed under the fluoroscope. Stoma edema may prevent visualization of the distal stomach and thereby delay prompt diagnosis of a distal perforation. Injection of contrast material through the nasogastric tube, if it crosses the anastomosis or gastrogastrostomy, can be very helpful. Contrast material should also be injected through a gastrostomy tube, if one is in place, to rule out a leak at this site or in the distal pouch. The patient must be examined in the upright and Trendelenburg positions. The latter assures complete filling of the fundus. Leaks can never be completely excluded unless a negative water-soluble contrast study is followed by a barium examination. Since surgery will follow promptly if a leak is demonstrated, we adjure the practice of doing only a water-soluble contrast study and sending the patient back to the unit. It takes only a few more minutes to complete the examination with barium. In one study, 17 of 30 upper gastrointestinal series were negative despite a free perforation.[33] Hence, exploration should be performed based on clinical signs and symptoms, even if all of the above investigations are negative. There is no real role for radionucleotide studies, in our opinion. In fact, even contrast studies may be unnecessary when a patient is obviously toxic without any other source of sepsis. Exploration is required whether the contrast study is positive or negative. However, such investigations may be helpful when time permits.

The intraoperative identification of the exact site of perforation may be difficult, and not infrequently the actual site is never found because of the tremendous phlegmon surrounding the stapled pouch. The earlier one operates, the easier it is to find and repair the hole. Later, primary closure is impossible and a tongue of omentum carefully fixed with nonabsorbable sutures must be used. Marlex mesh, if present, should be removed when possible, although we reported a gastric fistula which closed without removal of the Marlex.[53] A gastrostomy tube should be inserted into the distal stomach in GBP or into the fundus in GP.

For a leaking VBG, the anesthesiologist should try to position a nasogastric tube just above the channel, taking care not to enlarge the perforation. Edema may prevent identification of the GE junction, so the nasogastric tube may have to remain in the esophagus. Under such conditions, consideration should be given to a second gastrostomy inserted retrogradely into the smaller pouch. In this manner, a leak from the EEA staple line will be adequately drained. Even in the presence of intra-abdominal sepsis, these gastrostomies are safe if a long Witzel tunnel is fashioned using parietal peritoneum or omentum to seal their entrance sites and if the last hole is at least 4 inches into the stomach, with no pressure on the gastric wall from the tip of the tube. Similarly, one should not hesitate to insert a feeding jejunostomy. These patients will frequently have prolonged hospital courses, with the development of a gastric fistula. If sepsis continues, parenteral feeding may be difficult or impossible, and, in addition, enteral feeding may progress at home permitting earlier discharge.[53, 54] All abscess cavities are widely drained and debrided and soft drains placed through stab wounds, which must freely admit at least two fingers. The incision is closed with retention sutures and the skin left open unless contamination was minimal. One should take time to rule out a second perforation. Occasionally, surgeons have reported complete necrosis of the gastric pouch. This arises from ischemia or delayed diagnosis of a leak. In such cases, it is probably safer to perform a proximal esophagogastrectomy with an esophagogastric anastomosis through the abdominal incision (removing the xiphoid to aid exposure) rather than to take a chance with ongoing sepsis, which may lead to death. A cervical esophagostomy is a radical addition to be considered in some cases.

Efficacy of Gastric Partitioning

An analysis of the long-term success and failures for both GBP and GP must include an understanding of some basic concepts. Weight loss with both operations is greatest during the first 8–12 months, so that surgeons treating such patients tend to be very optimistic during this first year. However, there is a gradual reduction in the number of patients being followed up. After 1 year, results are difficult to interpret if one accepts the premise that a patient lost to follow-up may be losing weight inadequately or even regaining weight loss. Surgical conclusions should not be drawn until patients have been followed up for at least 2 years. There is a paucity of 3- to 5-year follow-up data, primarily because of constant changes in techniques. Many of us have performed operations on a series of patients, changed techniques, then performed operations on another series of patients, and so on. Hence, there is always a new variation, with follow-up rarely exceeding 2 years. One must ask if so many different surgical techniques have been introduced because the perfect surgical solution has not been found.

Mean weight loss with the original GBP was 35% of initial weight at 1 year, but no 5-year follow-up data have ever been published on these patients. In 1972, after 4 years of experience with GBP, GP came into vogue. At least 12 different variations were devised over the next 5 years. Thousands of HGP procedures were performed in university and community hospitals, yet it took more than 2 years to realize that this operation failed.[20]

The only prospective studies done show that at 2 years, GBP with Roux-en-Y is the most effective procedure, although even here, there is a paucity of 3- to 5-year data.[21, 55] Critical reviews of the literature show that most authors fail to include all of the necessary data for proper interpretation of results.[17, 21, 56] Follow-up is poor, and success or failure is not always defined. Series with 400–700 patients have less than 20% follow-up at 1 year.[57] When long-term data are given, it is seldom clear which patients are being reported. It is inadequate to give 24- and 36-month data without defining which patients are being followed up. Clearly only the best patients will be available for the longer follow-up. Expressing data in terms of "mean weight lost" is similarly misleading, since superheavyweights in the series will make results seem more favorable. However, percentage of weight lost or of excess weight, while more desirable, also has inherent flaws. A "mean percentage weight loss of 35%," while fitting the definition of "successful," means little if that patient weighed 500 pounds preoperatively. Probably the percentage of excess weight lost [= weight lost ÷ (preoperative − ideal weight)] is the best parameter since it compares the patient to himself, but multiple parameters must be used, including the absolute failure rates. For example, if two patients each weighing 300 pounds lost 50% (150 lb) and 10% (30 lb), respectively, after GP, "mean" percentage weight lost would be 30%, an acceptable figure, but the failure rate would be 50%.

Some authors who wrote extensively early in their experience did not update their data and this may very well indicate inadequate sustained weight loss. Gomez popularized one of the first reinforced HGP procedures, but only 24% of his first 200 patients were observed for 1 year.[58] Further follow-up data at 24 and 30 months did not indicate clearly the fate of the entire group, making determination of the failure rate difficult.[88]

Only 40 of 300 patients (13%) were followed up for 30 months. There are many other similar examples in the literature of 2- to 3-year follow-ups wherein only a small percentage of the initial group of patients were studied. For example, if only 10 of an initial 100 patients were available for follow-up at 3 years and all 10 had done well, the 3-year follow-up data would look good on paper but would not indicate what had happened to the other 90 patients. In series reporting adequate and sustained weight loss with HGP, one should also analyze the incidence of stoma obstruction. Favorable weight loss may reflect a number of miserable patients with tight gastrogastrostomies who can eat virtually nothing and require frequent hospital admissions for nutritional support and dilation. Finally, one must separate revisions from the rest of the group in order to properly assess success and failure rates. Clearly, a patient who requires a second operation is not a success.

Andersen et al. carried out a randomized trial of diet and GP compared with diet alone in 60 morbidly obese patients followed up for 2 years and found no differences in weight loss between the two groups.[59] However, the Gomez GP was used, and it is now appreciated that this operation will fail more than 75% of the time.[20] More prospective studies are needed.

With the appreciation that no variety of HGP can be efficacious, most surgeons either returned to Roux-en-Y GBP or switched to VBG. The latter is the simplest and safest procedure available to date. Mason reported 40 patients, 22 followed up for 6 months, who had two different stoma sizes, with an excess weight loss of 42%.[22] He sent to selected colleagues a report which updated his results. The patient data are combined with those from another center, each center using two different stoma diameters and grouping patients by their degrees of obesity. These data show patients losing from 30% to 70% of their excess weight at 2 years, but failure rates are not listed. We have been unable to find any other data published on VBG. Cautious optimism is justified, since the 1-year weight loss results compare favorably with GBP. The pessimist could argue that this lesser curve channel will eventually dilate as the Marlex gradually disrupts.

Since April 1982, we have performed 65 VBGs. Patients were assiduously followed in a special obesity clinic or by repeated telephone calls when necessary. Endoscopy and barium contrast studies were used to evaluate the pouch at 6-month intervals. Of the 46 patients, followed 6 months or longer, nine stopped losing weight before achieving a loss of at least 30% of body weight, five began to regain weight due to pouch dilation or staple disruption, and 13 are lost to follow-up. There were no early failures, in contrast to HGP, but the potential failure rate is at least 14 of 46 (30.5%) and could theoretically increase if the patients lost to follow-up prove to be failures. Hence, longer follow-up from all centers will be crucial to evaluate this procedure.

Failure to lose adequate weight after gastric partitioning procedures is related to dilation of the pouch or stoma, staple disruption, type of operation, and patient compliance.

As GP became technically easier and faster, more surgeons became interested in the procedure. In our center and others, dilation of the pouch itself or the narrow stoma was observed. This led to many technical variations designed to reinforce the stoma. Perhaps the ultimate failure of HGB could have been predicted from the earlier work of Printen and Mason, who described one variant of GP which they subsequently abandoned.[33, 60] Pace et al. were one of the first groups to present data on a highly simplified HGP. They applied a stapling device across the stomach and removed two staples, leaving a very narrow but unreinforced channel.[61] They operated on 220 patients in less than 2 years, of whom 119 were followed up for 1–4 months but only nine were available for 12-month follow-up. Cohn et al. used Pace's technique on 77 patients and noted a stabilized weight loss of only 20% of preoperative weight at 9 months. Ten patients failed to lose 10% of their weight, seven patients were lost to follow-up (these may well be failures), and there are no 2-year data.[62] Gomez, whose work was referred to above, reported on 300 patients in 1981. He claimed a 90% success rate, although only 13% of patients were followed up for 30 months and he did not include as failures patients who required revision (58.8%). This operation was widely practiced by many surgeons, all of whom had ultimately reported dismal results when patients were followed up 24 months or longer.[63] The entire GP field was reviewed by us.[20] That article was the first to point out that early, spectacular weight losses observed with this operation were not sustained. Patients followed up for 24 months or longer were frequently discovered to have regained much or all of the weight lost. Previously most surgeons cited failure rates of 25%–30%, which were acceptable and far superior to results obtained by conservative management. Other cautionary notes were issued by Jaffe, Halverson, the editors of *Lancet,* Moore, and Reinhold.[17, 63, 64, 66, 67] Halsted and Stern, summarizing a workshop on obesity treatment, concluded that surgical approaches cannot yet be judged successful and have largely led to the creation of new disease complexes affecting multiple organ systems.[65]

Smith performed three variations of GP on 200 patients and reported results in terms of pounds lost per month. The percentage of weight lost, the number of patients, length of follow-up, and individual failures were not given. Smith referred to 18-month follow-up data without stating how many patients were actually available for study. His graphs indicate that only nine patients were followed up for 15 months, yet he stated that "there has been no recurrence of weight gain."[68] Subsequently he updated his results, reporting "four year follow-ups" on 300 patients who had four different operations in 4 years.[69] He defined results in terms of pounds lost each month, without identifying how many patients were being studied. Even so, he cited a failure rate of 75% in the first two groups (84 patients). He stated that results were "good" or "excellent" in 70% of 193 patients with a reinforced HGP, and results were expressed as average weight loss (65 lb or 25% of body weight at 1 year). It was not clear how many patients were being followed up in this group. Despite his satisfaction, he switched to VBG.

Palombo et al. examined the weight lost in morbidly obese patients by measuring body composition.[70] The weight loss data showed that only 36 of 82 patients were available for 1-year follow-up studies and only 14 for 2-year follow-up.

MacLean et al. performed four types of GP in 79 patients.[71] In his series, as well as in many others, early dilation of the pouch and/or stoma led to technical changes, rendering assessment of long-term data difficult. To his credit, results were expressed in terms of the technical variation used. Maximum follow-up was 2 years, and 18 of 21 patients in groups 1 and 2 were failures. Follow-up of the 65 patients in groups 3 and 4 was less than 1 year. In 1983, MacLean et al. updated their data.[72] Results were good or satisfactory in 60% of patients with a mean follow-up of 28.5 months.

Thompson et al. operated on 150 carefully selected patients who were then followed up for 7–72 months postoperatively.[73] All patients had the same operation (loop GBP). This report stands alone with respect to the detailed analyses of complications and weight loss that are required. Only one patient was lost to follow-up. Thompson et al. have some of the best 3- to 5-year data reported to date for GBP, but even so only 46 of the original 150 patients have reached the 4-year follow-up mark (mean, 74% of excess weight lost), and the number of patients with inadequate weight loss is not stated.

Liner operated on 416 patients: 227 had GBP and 189 had HGP.[39] None of the latter were followed up more than 24 months. He reported a 50% failure rate, not including patients lost to follow-up.[74]

Dickerman operated on 39 patients using three different techniques. Three patients died, and the failure rate was at least 50%, with less than half the patients being followed up for more than 2 years.[75]

O'Leary devised yet another GP and published results in the first 35 patients.[76] The operative morbidity and mortality were "low" and weight loss was "adequate." There are no other data available for analysis.

Lechner and colleagues carried out one of the few well-controlled, prospective studies, first reported in 1981, with a recent updating of results.[77, 78] They reaffirmed the superiority of GBP over HGP for up to 36 months. Patients lost 74.1% vs. 62.0% of their excess weight at 36 months with GBP vs. HGP. However, only 24 of 221 patients were followed up for this period of time, and the number of failures was not given.

Herbst and Buckwalter reported on 7 years of experience in 292 patients who had four different operations. Complications occurred in 28% and reoperation was necessary in 18%. Weight loss was adequate as reported in all but one of the groups, but the number of patients lost to follow-up was not given, and the patients reported at 2 years were not individualized. No statements of patients with inadequate weight loss can be found.[79]

Many authors changed techniques during these developmental stages, including our group. This of itself is not serious, because the objective is to improve the operation. Of concern, however, is a lack of appreciation of the overall failure rate in a given center. A change in technique may lead to an improvement but does not excuse the researcher from his obligation to report the total number of patients operated on, listing all complications, individual failures, and patients lost to follow-up. He may then compare his latest technique with the overall (possibly poor) results to show that the change did or did not result in an improvement. Furthermore, it behooves the researchers to regularly update their data, indicating whether or not the initial results are valid at 3 or 4 years later.

It has been estimated that as of 1982, 25,000 patients had some form of GP in the United States (Joffe). In Canada, at least 5,000 procedures are being performed yearly. Therefore, it is important for interested surgeons to be updated. Mason initiated an annual obesity refresher course at the University of Iowa 8 years ago. In May 1983, the Bariatric Surgeons of Canada held the first National Symposium on the Surgical Treatment of Morbid Obesity, and the proceedings of this meeting will be published in the March and May issues of the *Canadian Journal of Surgery*. A second symposium will be held in May 1984. The University of Iowa course is held annually in June.

Staple Disruption

Staple line dehiscence can be partial or complete. In complete dehiscence, it is almost impossible to radiographically or endoscopically recognize that the stomach has ever been operated on.[80, 81] How this disruption occurs is not known, but the intake of solid food during the second to sixth week postoperatively has been implicated.[82] It is believed that disruption begins at the stoma and progresses laterally akin to the opening of a zipper. Dog experiments from our laboratory indicate that there is minimal fibrosis between the anterior and posterior gastric walls so that the bond is incomplete.[50] Linner had superior results when the staple line was reinforced by interrupted 00 silk sutures, suggesting that the inflammatory reaction to the silk helped create bridges across the staple line.[51] Ellison et al. were able to reduce the incidence of early staple line disruption from 30% to 6% by restricting the patients to a fluid diet for 8 weeks.[82] However, they found an increase in late failures from 18% in those who received solid food to 38% in those receiving a fluid diet, suggesting that fluid restriction merely delayed disruption or that hunger led the fluid-restricted patients to drink excessively. We keep patients NPO for 3–6 weeks, providing nutritional support by a feeding jejunostomy inserted routinely during GP. Oral intake progresses gradually from clear liquids at 1 ounce hourly, by measured medicine cups, to blenderized and then soft foods over 6 weeks. Meat and the skin of fish or poultry must be avoided for at least 6 months. Otherwise, troublesome obstructive symptoms will occur, leading to retching and increasing the chances of staple disruption.

There is a thick fat pad to the left of the esophagogastric junction which may prevent solid application of the staples, and we believe this should be removed. The stapling instrument should be held at right angles to the stomach. Ellison et al. measured the breaking strength of the staple line in dogs.[82] They found a significant correlation between the number of staples per inch of stomach and the strength of the staple line, especially during the first postoperative month, suggesting that the staples themselves contribute to the strength of the line. When staples disrupt, they often are pulled out from the posterior wall. If this occurs adjacent to the stoma only, the problem will resemble stoma dilation. Many of the technical variations of horizontal GP were developed to solve the problem of "stoma dilation" without a real appreciation that this was due to staple disruption. During repeated endoscopic examinations, we have observed staples, Prolene sutures, and Marlex in the lumen of the post-GP stomach.

Lechner and Elliott feel that the stomach must be crushed in order to create a fibrosed staple line. They use the smaller 3.5-mm rather than the 4.8-mm staples.[21] However, there is little objective data in this regard, and one could argue that the smaller staples might have more of a tendency to pull out.

Several authors have advocated the use of a suction gastrostomy inserted into the distal pouch to decrease the incidence of staple line disruption in GBP patients.[21]

Earlier HGPs were performed with a single row of staples. Nearly all of these patients experienced disruption of the staple lines, and most workers agree that two applications (four rows of staples) are required. The distance between the staples should be less than 0.5 cm or greater than 2.0 cm to avoid ischemia and possible perforation.[83] Occasionally, one of the two rows appears unsatisfactory and the surgeon is faced with the dilemma of whether or not to apply a third row of staples. We have found no objective data in this regard, but a third row has been used on several occasions by us without apparent misadventure. However, this should be used only when absolutely necessary.

Revisions

Revisions can be classified into early and late. Most of the former are for complications, including leaks, perforations, obstruction, and, occasionally, staple line dehiscence. Late revisions are usually necessary because of failure to lose adequate amounts of weight or regaining of weight lost. However, some reoperations are necessary because of stomal ulceration, bile reflux, or chronic stenoses. Unsatisfied or litigious patients complain of recurrent nausea, vomiting, and heartburn but the radiographic and gastroscopic appearance is normal. Paradoxically, many of these patients are actually gaining or at least losing inadequate amounts of weight. Their real problem lies in a subconscious desire to continue eating despite the inhibitions of their surgically created pouch. Reoperations in these patients, or for that matter in any patient who has had a GP, should be undertaken with great reservation. Previous devascularization and the dissection of the stomach from the diaphragm or liver may lead to many postoperative complications, and the mortality ranges from 2% to 4%. It is always difficult to separate the technical failures from those caused by noncompliant patients. In the latter instance, the risks of revision are simply not justified.[63, 84] Data from the surgical literature are weak regarding revisions. Frequently, revisions are not separated in the data analysis. This is important, because a patient who requires revision must by definition be a "failure." Moreover, long-term data showing the exact percentage of patients revised who actually benefit from sustained weight loss are unavailable.

Stomal Ulcers

The incidence of stomal ulceration after GBP varies from 1.8% to 3.1%.[33, 85] Mason and Ito demonstrated in animals that a two-thirds gastric exclusion was not ulcerogenic. If the staple or transection level was too low, a large part of the acid-producing part of the stomach (above the staples) is excluded, thereby bathing the distal stomach with alkaline juice. This is essentially an antral exclusion procedure. The problem has become less common with appreciation of the need for a small proximal gastric pouch.[86, 87] In fact, stomal ulceration in a GBP with a pouch of less than 50 ml indicates a probable underlying ulcer diathesis. Certainly the incidence of stomal ulceration is not high enough to warrant routine vagotomy as part of the initial procedure. Older patients seem more susceptible to stomal ulceration. The problem seems to be nonexistent with GP unless there is an underlying ulcer diathesis.

The surgeon will occasionally encounter an obese patient with a peptic ulcer. It is tempting to consider simultaneous vagotomy, pyloroplasty, and GP, but such a combined procedure is of unproved clinical merit. The clinical findings in stomal ulceration included persistent pain, vomiting, and bleeding, especially without evidence of stoma obstruction to explain the vomiting. Stomal ulceration may also be manifested by unexplained anemia or frank hemorrhage.[89] Isolated cases of antral perforation years after the GBP procedure have been reported.[90]

Since stomal ulceration is caused by either too large a proximal pouch or an underlying ulcer diathesis, the therapeutic alternatives are either to reduce the size of the proximal pouch (usually by simple amputation using stapling instruments), to perform an antiulcer operation, or to take down the GBP and convert it to a GP. The possibility of an underlying ulcer diathesis must always be kept in mind, whether dealing with a new patient or when faced with the necessity for reoperation. At worst, the patient's ulcer might not heal. Therefore, the question must be asked: what reoperation would be done in a patient with a GP or GBP if vagotomy and drainage failed and gastric resection were necessary? When vagotomy is required, it is more reasonable to consider the truncal type because the blood supply along the lesser curve must be preserved to nourish the upper pouch. If a stomal ulcer occurs in a patient who has a pouch of not more than 100 ml, treatment with cimetidine and antacids should suffice.[88]

Stoma Obstruction

Stoma size is more important in GP than GBP. If there is an increase in stoma size, the GP patient fails to lose weight, whereas GBP patients simply dump. Notwithstanding the apparent superiority of GBP over GP, many surgeons performing the former now reinforce the gastrojejunal anastomosis. Perhaps the most common manifestation of stomal dysfunction is a sensation of substernal fullness and possible heartburn in the early postoperative period. The esophagus may be grossly dilated. All of these signs and symptoms usually resolve with time and with supportive care using antacids, meat tenderizer, Maxeran, and a liquid to soft diet.

Reinforcement of GP stomas has preoccupied surgeons for nearly 8 years. If the stoma is larger than 12 mm, weight loss will eventually prove inadequate. Conversely, attempts to reduce the stoma to less than 8 mm or to reinforce it with external Marlex or sutures led to a significant incidence of stoma obstruction and reoperations. Some stenoses appear early and are related to the actual size of the internal lumen created during the procedure. Late obstructions, even when the internal lumen has been carefully calibrated, are probably related to mucosal injury secondary to crushing during application of the stapler. Alternatively, late stenoses may be secondary to scar contraction which in turn arose from a subclinical leak. Those who reinforce staple lines with through-and-through silk sutures have been bothered with stenoses.

Gomez tried to solve the problem of mucosal crushing by using a C clamp during horizontal application of the stapler.[58] However, since horizontal GP has now been abandoned, this maneuver is no longer required, and of course the mucosa is not crushed during VBG. It is felt that the incidence of stoma obstruction is declining with the move over to VBG. This stoma is carefully calibrated and limitation of its diameter is achieved by the external application of Marlex around a 32 French tube. Also, the stoma, which is on the lesser curve, is much easier to dilate if obstruction does occur.

Perhaps the most important surgical principle in dealing with stoma obstruction is to appreciate that in most of these patients, the tight stomas will dilate with time. Conservativism is the key and reoperation is seldom necessary. In our series of 172 patients with GP, 32 (18%) developed stoma stenosis, defined as an inability to drink fluids and/or swallow saliva. All were managed conservatively in the hospital or as outpatients. Management consisted of total parenteral nutrition and endoscopy to evaluate the stoma with or without dilation using Eder-Puestow dilators and long-term enteral nutrition through a feeding jejunostomy. Of 32 patients, 13 were dilated, in a total of 36 procedures, up to the maximum size (45 French). Twenty-nine required repletion by combined parenteral and enteral nutrition. Three required jejunostomy insertion as a separate procedure. Patients were followed up 6–60 months. Thirty-one did well. Gastrogastrostomy was required in one patient with a stenosis following a second GP. Two dilated patients actually regained to weights 40% over ideal. These data indicate that reoperation is seldom needed, no matter how severe the stenosis. Long-term outpatient enteral feeding is of extreme value since the temptation to operate is much greater if the patient is in the hospital. Insertion of a feeding jejunostomy, even as a separate procedure, permits treatment at home as well as temporization of reoperation.[91]

Patients presenting with acute obstruction may have food or gelatin capsules caught in the stoma. Careful instructions prior to discharge will prevent the majority of these problems. Admission is seldom necessary if a feeding jejunostomy has been inserted. The patient merely remains NPO and takes meat tenderizer or Papain orally to dissolve the obstructing particle. Endoscopy with a pediatric instrument will successfully dislodge the bezoar if conservative treatment fails and at the same time permits evaluation of the stoma.

Reflux

Dogs with GBP and a loop gastroenterostomy develop diffuse erythematous esophagitis without ulceration consistent with bile reflux.[33] When a Roux-en-y loop was used instead of a loop gastroenterostomy, no esophageal mucosal abnormalities were detected. This suggests that bile reflux is related to the type of gastrojejunostomy performed, and clinical data in patients having GBP confirm this experimental evidence.[92, 95] Bile and acid are equally important in the genesis of esophagitis. With respect to GBP, there is no need to be concerned about acid reflux if the pouch is less than 50 ml. Similarly, bile esophagitis will not occur if a Roux-en-y gastrojejunostomy is performed. Patients with documented gastroesophageal reflux need not have antireflux procedures in conjunction with GBP, partially because of the above. Also, weight loss by itself is therapeutic with respect to reflux—an extremely common problem in any patient who exceeds ideal weight by 30% or more. An antireflux procedure would interfere with the blood supply to the small fundic pouch, and if both a GBP or GP and an antireflux procedure are performed simultaneously, there is a risk of creating a closed segment which is prone to rupture postoperatively.

Reflux esophagitis in the long-term predisposes to the development of Barret's esophagitis with an increased risk of malignancy. Reflux gastritis may be relatively asymptomatic. It is known that intestinal contents will cause more severe gastritis than bile or pancreatic secretions alone. Injury to the mucosal barrier increases permeability to acid and other substances such as ingested carcinogens. With GBP, the reduced acidity in the proximal pouch combined with gastritis is reminiscent of the known risk of carcinoma developing in the pouch of patients who had high subtotal gastrectomies for ulcer disease.[93, 94] The long-term malignant potential of GBP has not yet been assessed.

Summary

Death rates for the morbidly obese are at least 11 times higher than for the nonobese, although the most popular and frequently cited study involved men only.[3] In addition to the risk of disease, morbidly obese patients are subject to social and economic discrimination. This severely impairs their ability to function in society. The benefits from weight loss include frequent amelioration of complications, such as hypertension, cardiorespiratory disease, diabetes, and so forth. But a reduction in the mortality with weight loss has not yet been demonstrated, and many obese patients are in apparent good health for years.

Surgery seems to offer the only hope for these unfortunate patients, but it is important to avoid overenthusiastic approaches until long-term, prospective studies clearly establish efficacy and unsuspected complications. The literature suffers from short follow-up periods and lack of standardization of the operative procedure. Various methods of reporting results have made comparison and interpretation difficult.[17, 63, 64, 66, 67, 73]

. . . . from an ethical and moral aspect, all of these operations are being abused. Too many are being done on patients who are not valid candidates and by surgeons unqualified or without adequate follow-up programs. This malignant abuse could result in discreditation of the surgical approach and lead to abandonment of the only practical method for treating morbid obesity. . . ."[17]

We, as responsible surgeons, must strive to achieve the highest possible quality and accuracy in the analysis and presentation of our data. Guidelines have been reviewed herein. The importance of regular subspecialty meetings for bariatric surgeons cannot be overemphasized. Registries are essential in order to quickly and accurately disseminate information as it becomes available. All of these procedures are in the developmental stages and should only be performed by surgeons with the capabilities of following the patients for long periods of time. Editors of journals could help by either accepting or modifying criteria for publication of bariatric surgical data and by using these criteria to assist authors in the preparation of their manuscripts.

REFERENCES

1. Dublin L.I., Jimenis A.O., Marks H.H.: Factors in the selection of risks with a history of gallbladder disease. *Trans. Assoc. Life Insur. Med. Dir. Am.* 21:34, 1934.
2. Rimm A.A., Werner L.H., Bernstein R., et al.: Disease and obesity in 73,532 women. *Obes. Bariatr. Med.* 1:77, 1972.
3. Drenick E.J., et al.: Excessive mortality and causes of death in morbidly obese men. *JAMA* 243:443, 1980.
4. Gordon T., Kanel W.B.: Obesity and cardiovascular diseases: The Framingham Study. *Clin. Endocrinol. Metabol.* 5:367, 1976.
5. Van Itallie T.B.: Obesity: Adverse effects on health and longevity. *Am. J. Clin. Nutr.* 32:2723, 1979.
6. Strauss R.J., Wise L.: Operative risks of obesity. *Surg. Gynecol. Obstet.* 146:286–291, 1978.
7. Pemberton L.B., Manax W.G.: Relationship of obesity to postop complications after cholecystectomy. *Am. J. Surg.* 121:110, 1971.
8. Postlethwait R.W., Johnson W.D.: Complications following surgery for duodenal ulcer in obese patients. *Arch. Surg.* 105:448, 1972.
9. Stunkard A.: Behavior modification in the treatment of obesity, in Bray G.A., Bethune J.E. (eds.): *Treatment and Management of Obesity.* New York, Harper & Row, 1974, pp. 103–116.

10. Penick S.B., Stunkard A.J.: The treatment of obesity. *Adv. Psychosom. Med.* 7:217, 1972.
11. Stunkard A.J., McLaren H.M.: The results of treatment for obesity. *Arch. Intern. Med.* 102:79, 1959.
12. National Institutes of Health Consensus Development Conference on Surgical Treatment of Morbid Obesity. *Ann. Surg.* 185:189–455, 1979.
13. Kannel W.B., Gordon T.: Physiological and medical concomitants of obesity: The Framingham Study, in Bray G.A. (ed.): *Obesity in America.* NIH publication No. 179–359, 1979, pp. 125–163.
14. Rabkin S.W., Mathewson F.A.L., Hsu P.H.: Relationship of body weight to development of ischemic heart disease in a cohort of young North American men after 26 years' observation period: The Manitoba Study. *Am. J. Cardiol.* 39:452, 1977.
15. Printen K.J., Mason E.E.: Gastric bypass for morbid obesity in patients more than fifty years of age. *Surg. Gynecol. Obstet.* 144:192, 1977.
16. Freeman J.B., Masters R.G.: Surgery for morbid obesity, in Yarborough M.F. and Curreri W.P. (eds.): *Surgical Nutrition,* vol. 3. New York, Churchill Livingstone, Inc., 1981.
17. Jaffe S.N.: A review: Surgery for morbid obesity. *J. Surg. Res.* 33:74, 1982.
18. DenBesten L., Kuchenbecker S.: *Metabolic surgery for obesity.* Chicago, Year Book Medical Publishers, Inc., 1980.
19. Mason E.E., Ito C.C.: Gastric bypass. *Ann. Surg.* 170:329, 1969.
20. Freeman J.B., Burchett H.: Escalating failure rate with gastric partitioning for morbid obesity. *Am. J. Surg.* 145:113–119, 1983.
21. Lechner G.W., Elliott D.W.: Comparison of weight loss after gastric exclusion and partitioning. *Arch. Surg.* 118:685–692, 1983.
22. Mason E.E.: Vertical banded gastroplasty. *Arch. Surg.* 117:701, 1982.
23. Flanagan L.: Controlling the size of the gastrojejunostomy stoma in gastric bypass operations. *Surg. Gynecol. Obstet.* 157:377, 1983.
24. Scopinaro N., et al.: Biliopancreatic bypass for obesity. *Br. J. Surg.* 66:618, 1980.
25. Rochester D.F., Enson Y.: Current concepts in the pathogenesis of the obesity-hypoventilation syndrome: Mechanical and circulatory factors. *Am. J. Med.* 57:402–419, 1974.
26. Anesthesia and the obese patient, in Brown B.R. Jr. (ed.): *Contemporary Anesthesia Practice.* Philadelphia, F.A. Davis Co., 1982.
27. Young S.R., et al. Anesthetic biotransformation of renal function in obese patients during and after methoxyflurane or halothane anesthesia. *Anesthesiology* 42:451–457, 1975.
28. Randall C.C., et al.: General anesthesia for morbidly obese patients: An examination of postoperative outcomes. *Anesthesiology* 54:310–313, 1981.
29. King G.E.: Errors in clinical measurements of blood pressure in obesity. *Clin. Sci.* 32:223–237, 1967.
30. Vaughan R.W., Wise L.: Choice of abdominal operative incision in the obese patient: A study using blood gas measurements. *Ann. Surg.* 181:829–835, 1975.
31. Fox G.S., Whalley O.G., Bevan O.R.: Anaesthesia for the morbidly obese: Experience with 110 patients. *Br. J. Anaesthes.* 53:811–816, 1981.

32. Paul D.R., Hoyt J.L., Boutras A.R.: Cardiovascular and respiratory changes in response to change of posture in the very obese. *Anesthesiology* 45:73–78, 1976.
33. Mason E.E.: *Surgery for Morbid Obesity. Major Problems in Clinical Surgery*, vol. 26. Philadelphia, W.B. Saunders Co., 1981.
34. Joseph A., et al.: Perioperative complications of gastric restrictive operations. *Am. J. Surg.* 146:613–618, 1983.
35. Pories W.J., et al.: Prophylactic cephazolin in gastric bypass surgery. *Surgery* 90:426–432, 1981.
36. Hamilton D.L., et al.: Liver injury with alcoholic-like hyalin after gastroplasty for morbid obesity. *Gastroenterology* 85:722–726, 1983.
37. Mason E.E., et al.: Gastric bypass in morbid obesity. *Am. J. Clin. Nutr.* 33:395–405, 1980.
38. Buckwalter J.A.: Clinical trial of jejuno-ileal and gastric bypass for the treatment of morbid obesity: Four years' progress report. *Am. J. Surg.* 46:377–381, 1980.
39. Sassaris M., et al.: Neuropsychiatric syndromes after gastric partition. *Am. J. Gastroenterol.* 78:321–323, 1983.
40. Feit H., et al.: Peripheral neuropathy and starvation after gastric partitioning for morbid obesity. *Ann. Intern. Med.* 96:453, 1982.
41. Haid R.W., et al.: Wernicke-Korsakoff encephalopathy after gastric plication. *JAMA* 247:2566–2567, 1982.
42. Printen K.J., Mason E.E.: Peripheral neuropathy following gastric bypass for the treatment of morbid obesity. *Obes. Bariatr. Med.* 6:185, 1977.
43. Nutritional complications of surgical treatment of morbid obesity. *Nutr. Rev.* 38:238, 1980.
44. MacLean L.D.: *Can. J. Surg.*, to be published.
45. Crowley L.V., Olson R.W.: Megaloblastic anemia after gastric bypass for obesity. *Am. J. Gastroenterol.* 78:406–410, 1983.
46. Schneider S.B., et al.: Cutaneous anergy and marrow suppression as complications of gastroplasty for morbid obesity. *Surgery* 94:109, 1983.
47. Cogbill T.H., et al.: Perforation after gastric partitioning for morbid obesity. *Surgery* 92(3):551–552, 1982.
48. Mason E.E., et al.: Risk reduction in gastric operations for obesity. *Ann. Surg.* 190(2):158–165, 1979.
49. Printen K.J., et al.: Increasing the efficacy of gastric operations for the control of morbid obesity. *Am. Surg.* 48:309–313, 1982.
50. Gudas V, Freeman J.B.: Canine gastroplasty experiments involving incorporation of mesh into staple lines. *Am. Surg.* 48:44, 1982.
51. Linner J.H.: Comparative effectiveness of gastric bypass and gastroplasty. *Arch. Surg.* 117:695–700, 1982.
52. Beisel W.R., Wannemacher R.W.: Gluconeogenesis, ureagenesis and ketogenesis during sepsis. *JPEN* 4:277–285, 1980.
53. MacMillan I., Freeman J.B.: Closure of a gastric fistula in the presence of Marlex. *Can. J. Surg.*, to be published.
54. Freeman J.B., Fairfull-Smith R.: Feeding jejunostomy. *Can. J. Surg.*, 1981.
55. Griffen W.O., et al.: A prospective comparison of gastric and jejuno-ileal bypass procedures for morbid obesity. *Surgery* 186:500, 1977.

56. Reinhold R.B.: Critical analysis of long term weight loss following gastric bypass. *Surg. Gynecol. Obstet.* 155:385–394, 1982.
57. Murphy K., McCracken J.D., Ozment K.L.: Gastric bypass for obesity: Results of a community hospital series. *Am. J. Surg.* 140:747–750, 1980.
58. Gomez C.A.: Gastroplasty in the surgical management of morbid obesity. *Am. J. Clin. Nutr.* 33:406–415, 1980.
59. Andersen T., Backer O., et al.: Randomized trial of diet and gastroplasty compared with diet alone in morbid obesity. *N. Engl. J. Med.* 310:352–356, 1984.
60. Printen J.G., Mason E.E.: Gastric bypass for relief of morbid obesity. *Arch. Surg.* 106:428, 1973.
61. Pace W.G., et al.: Gastric partitioning for morbid obesity. *Ann. Surg.* 190:392, 1979.
62. Cohn R., et al.: Gastric stapling for morbid obesity. *Am. J. Surg.* 142:67, 1981.
63. Halverson J.D.: Obesity surgery in perspective. *Surgery* 87:119, 1980.
64. Editorial. *Lancet* 1:1275, 1979.
65. National Institutes of Health Concensus Development Conference on Surgical Treatment of Morbid Obesity. *Ann. Surg.* 189:455, 1979.
66. Moore E.E., et al.: Gastric bypass operations: Surgical pros and cons. *Surg. Gynecol. Obstet.* 148:764, 1979.
67. Reinhold R.B.: Critical analysis of long term weight loss following gastric bypass. *Surg. Gynecol. Obstet.* 155:385–394, 1982.
68. Smith L.B.: Modification of the gastric partitioning procedure for morbid obesity. *Am. J. Surg.* 142:725, 1981.
69. Smith L.B., et al.: Results and complications of gastric partitioning: Four-year follow-up of 300 morbidly obese patients. *Am. J. Surg.* 146:815–819, 1983.
70. Palombo J.D., et al.: Composition of weight loss in morbidly obese patients after gastric bypass. *J. Surg. Res.* 30:435, 1981.
71. MacLean L.D., et al.: Gastroplasty for obesity. *Surg. Gynecol. Obstet.* 153:200, 1981.
72. Maclean L.D., et al.: Nutrition following gastric operations for morbid obesity. *Ann. Surg.* 196:347–355, 1983.
73. Thompson W.R., et al.: Complications and weight loss in 150 consecutive gastric exclusion patients: Critical review. *Am. J. Surg.* 146:602–612, 1983.
74. Liner J.: Comparative effectiveness of gastric bypass and gastroplasty. *Arch. Surg.* 117:965, 1982.
75. Dickerman R.M.: Gastric exclusion surgery in the management of morbid obesity. *Annu. Rev. Med.* 33:263–270, 1982.
76. O'Leary J.P.: Partition of the lesser curvature of the stomach in morbid obesity. *Surg. Gynecol. Obstet.* 154:85–86, 1982.
77. Lechner G.W., Callender A.K.: Subtotal gastric exclusion and gastric partitioning: A randomized prospective comparison of one hundred patients. *Surgery* 90:637, 1981.
78. Lechner G.W., Elliott D.W.: Comparison of weight loss after gastric exclusion and partitioning. *Arch. Surg.* 118:685–692, 1983.

79. Herbst C.A., Buckwalter J.A.: Weight loss and complications after four gastric operations for morbid obesity. *South. Med. J.* 75:1324–1328, 1982.
80. Aghn F.P., et al.: Gastroplasty for morbid obesity: Roentgen evaluation and spectrum of complications. *Gastrointest. Radiol.* 7:217–223, 1983.
81. Hammond D.I., Freeman J.B.: Radiology of gastroplasty for morbid obesity. *J. Can. Assoc. Radiol.* 33:21–24, 1982.
82. Ellison E.C., et al.: Prevention of early failure of stapled gastric partitions in treatment of morbid obesity. *Arch. Surg.* 115:528–533, 1981.
83. Printen K.J., et al.: Increasing the efficacy of gastric operations for the control of morbid obesity. *Am. Surg.* 48:309–313, 1982.
84. Halverson J.D., Koehler R.E.: Assessment of patients with failed gastric operations for morbid obesity. *Am. J. Surg.* 145:357–363, 1983.
85. Mason E.E., et al.: Optimizing results of gastric bypass. *Ann. Surg.* 182:405–414, 1975.
86. Printen K.J., et al.: Stomal ulcers after gastric bypass. *Arch. Surg.* 115:525, 1980.
87. Mason E.E., Printen K.J.: Gastric bypass for obesity, in Buchwald H., Varco L. (eds.): *Metabolic Surgery.* New York, Grune & Stratton, 1978, pp. 41–57.
88. Gomez C.A.: Gastroplasty in intractable obesity. *Int. J. Obesity* 5:413–420, 1981.
89. Printen K.J., et al.: Bleeding for the bypassed stomach following gastric bypass. *Surg. Gynecol. Obstet.* 156:65, 1983.
90. Anderson O.S., et al.: An unusual complication of gastric bypass: Perforated antral ulcer. *Am. J. Gastroenterol.* 77:93–94, 1982.
91. AlHalees Z., Freeman J.B.: Conservative management of post-gastroplasty obstruction. *JPEN* 8:95, 1984.
92. Griffen W.O., et al.: Gastric bypass for morbid obesity. *World J. Surg.* 5:817–822, 1981,
93. Pygott F., Shaf V.S.: Gastric cancer associated with gastroenterostomy and partial gastrectomy. *Gut* 9:117, 1968.
94. Domellof L., et al.; Late pre-Cancerous changes in carcinoma of the gastric stump after Billroth I resection. *Am. J. Surg.* 132:26, 1976.
95. Delaney J.P., et al.: Pyloric reflux gastritis: The offending agent. *Surgery* 77:764, 1975.

Subject Index